Introduction

Ketogenic diets, or keto diets, are one of the latest health and lifestyle trends that took the internet by storm. It is characterized by low carbs, medium protein, and high-fat consumption. It may sound strange and counterintuitive, but keto diets have been linked to weight loss and other mental and physical benefits to both young and old people alike.

It is no hogwash pseudoscience either because many studies have been done on the subject and they all agree that keto diets work. But how exactly do they work and how you can get started? Read more to find out.

Ketogenic Diet and Aging

There are many scientific theories out there that explain how the human body ages and deteriorates over time, two of which are free radical theory of aging and glycation theory of aging.

The free radical theory explains that our body becomes damaged because of the free radicals trying to bind to the molecules in our body in their search for more electron, which leads to damage and inflammation. In the process of binding, your molecule becomes unstable and binds with your other molecule to get its electron, and the cycle repeats in a process known as oxidation, causing a lot of damage over time. The solution this theory proposed is to increase your body's pool of antioxidants because they have an extra electron to give to the free radicals in your body, thus preventing them from taking and destabilizing your body's molecules.

The glycation theory of aging proposes that we age because of the glycation damage from high blood sugar. That means the excess sugar in the body clings onto the proteins in the body, preventing them from doing their jobs, which can lead to many complications, one of which is diabetes.

But how does the keto diet come in? Keto diets can help the body slow the aging process in many ways:

1. Keto diet minimizes damages done by oxidation and increases the body's store of uric acid and other antioxidants.
2. Ketosis increases the mitochondrial glutathione, which is a potent antioxidant that resides within the mitochondria, the powerhouse of your cell. Antioxidants that are digested orally are not very effective in protecting your cells. But ketosis supports the cell directly.
3. Keto diets are very low in sugar, meaning that your blood sugar level would be much lower, reducing the chance of glycation damages.
4. Keto diets are low in carbs, which improves blood sugar control level and suppress appetite because they have the same effects as fasting.
5. Keto diets also reduce triglycerides, which are the fatty acids in

the bloodstream that are used to measure heart disease risk. You want triglycerides in your body to be as low as possible.

In short, keto diets reduce your blood sugar level, prevent glycation damages, and inflammation. These three conditions are associated with all sorts of diseases that lead to death. Therefore, keto diets ate the best way to reduce blood sugar and insulin levels, increase your longevity and wellbeing.

The Science Behind Keto

Okay, so we know that a ketogenic diet is characterized by low-carb, medium-protein, and high-fat intake. The combination of these three ingredients will cause the body to go into ketosis. Ketosis is a metabolic shift in the body in a way that allows the body to burn fat rather than carbohydrates.

The carbohydrates that are consumed are converted into glucose and insulin. Here, glucose is basically sugar. Glucose is the most convenient source of energy because your body can convert it to energy easier. As such, the body prefers using that up first. Another byproduct of carbohydrates is insulin, which is a hormone produced by your pancreas. This hormone helps process glucose in your body by transporting the glucose in the body to where it is needed. When your body has enough energy, the excess glucose will be converted to adipose tissue, or fat, as a backup. Of course, that does not mean that the body uses that fat first if there are carbohydrates available.

You see, the fat in your body is considered to be the backup source of power. Therefore, in a normal situation, your body would burn carbohydrates, then fats, then proteins, in that order. As such, the body does not burn fat as effectively. Ketosis promotes weight loss by making the body prioritize burning fat, thus resulting in more fat being burned.

Many ordinary diets contain plenty of carbohydrates, which are not bad in itself. It is only bad when you take in more energy than you spend it, which means you create an energy leftover which would be converted to fat. Day by day, your weight adds up very quickly. For such a diet, glucose is the main source of energy because it contains plenty of it. However, the glucose in your body can only last you a few days. Your body will convert glucose to fat if you do not use glucose up. So when your glucose store runs dry in a few days, your body will switch to another source of energy through a biochemical process known as ketogenesis.

When this process starts, your liver starts to take the fat in your body and break it down, creating an alternative source of energy. When that happens, your ketone level goes up and your body. This is the moment when you enter ketosis.

How to Enter Ketosis

You have a few options when it comes to entering ketosis.

The most direct one is by depriving your body of carbohydrates, therefore glucose, through fasting for a long period of time. When you stop eating altogether, your body will turn to burn fat as a source of energy because it has no glucose to work with. But of course, fasting and intermittent fasting is a whole different subject on its own and we will not cover that in this book. But do remember that fasting has its caveat.

Another option is to eat less. You just have to consume less than 20 to 50 grams of your daily carbohydrate intake a day. This will depend on who is fasting. Some require fewer while some require more, perhaps even more than 50 grams. However, the bottom line is that people who are on a keto diet only consume 5% of their usual carbohydrate intake.

But whatever method you use, it all boils down to this:

1. Cut down on carbs intake to 5% of regular intake
2. Increase fat intake to 80%
3. The lack of carbs will force the body to burn fat instead
4. When the ketone level in your blood rises high enough, you enter a state of ketosis
5. Profit.

Benefits

Keto diet is unlike any other diet that disappears just as abruptly as they appear. In fact, the keto diet has been practiced for far longer than you think. Its root can be traced back to the 1920s. A ketogenic diet is based on a solid understanding of physiology and nutrition science, so it is not some hogwash pseudoscience either. It is grounded on science and it has been proven to be effective.

Keto diet is very effective for many people because it provides a wide variety of benefits that anyone can benefit from, regardless of their gender or age. Some of the benefits are the direct remedy to weight gain such as hormonal imbalance (especially for menopause), elevated insulin as well as high blood sugar level. A keto diet is not only beneficial for the body either. The diet has therapeutic benefits that really help those who have brain disorders.

Weight Loss

Of course, the main reason why people jump on the keto wagon in the first place is the fact that the keto diet is an effective way to lose weight. A diet that is rich in fat content but low in carbs such as the keto diet minimizes hunger in your body. It just does not feel as hungry when you are in ketosis. Not only that, but your body's ability to burn fat is also boosted due to hormonal changes in your body.

When you eat normally by following an ordinary diet, the food you eat provides your body with carbohydrates. When they enter the system, your body releases insulin. Insulin helps regulate blood sugar levels by converting the excess into fat for later use. With a lower level of insulin, our body is more likely to use existing fat in the body for energy instead of storing the excess energy as fat.

Moreover, a keto diet that packs a lot of healthy fat and protein is very filling, which can help suppress your appetite and prevent overeating.

Cholesterol and Blood Pressure

Diabetes and high blood pressure are some of the most common reasons that result in death among older adults. Keto diet is effective in this regard because it improves triglyceride and cholesterol levels that are associated with arterial buildups. It also leads to an increase in high-density lipoprotein (HDL) and decreases in low-density lipoprotein (LDL) particles. All of this comes together to the improvement in blood pressure.

But high blood pressure can also result from cholesterol in the body, which is a consequence of excess weight.

Regulate Blood Sugar

Keto diet helps regulate blood sugar by controlling how much insulin is in the system. Maintaining the right level of insulin is important because you can avoid problems such as insulin resistance or pre-diabetes. Keto diet has also been shown to reduce HbA1c levels, which is a measure of blood glucose control.

Because the keto diet is effective at regulating insulin, therefore blood sugar level, it has an added benefit of helping people with type 2 diabetes. It may not cure them outright, but it can work in conjunction with diabetes medication or reduce its dependence.

Fights Neurological Disorders

Keto diet has been used in the past to treat neurological disorders or other cognitive impairments such as epilepsy. When your body goes into ketosis, your body produces ketones that help reverse neurodegenerative illnesses. Here, the brain just uses another source of energy instead of using the cellular energy pathway that is faulty in people with brain disorders. That means the keto diet can help prevent or treat disorders such as Parkinson's and Alzheimer's.

How to Get Started with the Ketogenic Diet When You're Over 50?

Jumping on the keto wagon, as well as committing to anything, can be an intimidating endeavor. However, getting started with this is relatively simple. No matter how many forms of the keto diet that are out there, they share some similarities:

Restrict Carbohydrates: This is the entire point of a keto diet – little carbs intake. A keto diet should have less than 20g of net carbs a day, although some people can go up to 30g. If you can get this right, then you are well on your way to become successful in your ketogenic diet adventure. Other than that, there are a few more things to keep in mind:

1. Limit protein intake: A keto diet consists mostly of fat, not carbs or protein. Too much protein can put undue stress on your kidneys and the excess will be converted to glucose, then stored as fat anyway. So make sure that you get your protein portion just right as well. This should be the second priority after setting your daily carbs limit.

2. Use fat as a lever: Fat isn't necessarily a bad thing, especially in a keto diet because fat makes up a huge portion of your keto diet. This is because fat is both a source of energy and satiety. Here, fat serves as a lever in your keto diet whereas carbs and protein remain constant. That means you can determine how much weight you want to gain or lose based on how much fat you consume. Because our goal is to lose weight, that means you need to eat just enough fat. No more, no less.

3. Drink water: Water is very important in a keto diet because your body needs it to store glycogen in the liver. When you eat foods low in carbs, the body uses up glycogen so you can burn fat, which also means depleting your water store as well. That means you will become dehydrated faster. You normally need 2 gallons a day, but I recommend going up to 3 or 4 gallons a day when you are on a keto diet.

4. Take care of the electrolytes: Potassium, sodium, and magnesium

are the major electrolytes in the body. Since a keto diet uses up water in the body, that also means that the electrolytes go along with the water. When you do not have enough electrolytes in the body, you feel sick. This is commonly referred to as the "keto flu". Although this is only temporary, you do not have to suffer the keto fly if you keep your electrolytes level at a sufficient level. That means salting your food, drinking bone broth or any other broth, and eating picked veggies. If any of these alternatives are unfavorable for you, you can also take supplements to top up your electrolytes store, but make sure you consult your doctor first before you do that.

5. Eat when you are hungry: Only when you are hungry, then eat. Some people have the mindset that they need to eat at least 4 to 6 meals, or even snack constantly between mealtimes. No wonder why they gain weight so much. In a keto diet, frequent eating is not recommended as it can interfere with your weight loss effort. So eat only when you are hungry. If you do not feel hungry, then don't eat. But this should be easy considering that a keto diet or any other low-carb diets lack carbohydrate so this diet naturally suppresses appetite altogether.

6. Focus on whole foods: You do not have to resort to eating only natural or whole food so you can get your carbs limit down properly. However, keep in mind that processed food is rich in carbs and will not help you get rid of cravings, not to mention that they are unhealthy in the first place.

7. Exercise: This is optional, but you should take care of your muscles at your age as they start to degrade. You will feel better, your health will improve, and your weight will go down faster.

Keto Macro

If you really want to get it down, you will need an online calculator to help you determine how much you need to eat. It is impossible to give you a direct formula because there are many variables to take into consideration. But if you are curious, a keto diet usually contains the following:

- Fat: 60% to 75%

- Protein: 15% to 30%
- Net carbs: 5% to 10%

Fat, protein and net carbs content vary from person to person, but they all stay within this range. It is worth mentioning that the sum of all three should equal 100%. The percentage is the amount of daily calorie intake.

Best Foods to Fit into the Keto Diet for Older Adults

In this chapter, I will go over what food you should consider incorporating into your keto diet. But the general guideline is that all foods that are nutritious and low in carbs are excellent options.

Seafood

Fishes and shellfishes are perfect for keto diets. Many fishes are rich in B vitamins, potassium, as well as selenium. Salmon, sardines, mackerel, and other fatty fish also pack a lot of omega-3 fats that help in regulating insulin levels. These are so low in carbs that it is negligible.

Shellfishes are a different story because some contain very few carbs whereas others pack plenty. Shrimps and most crabs are okay but beware of other types of shellfish.

Vegetables

Most vegetables pack a lot of nutrients that your body can greatly benefit from even though they are low in calories and carbs. Plus, some of them contain fiber, which helps with your bowel movement. Moreover, your body spends more energy breaking down and digesting food rich in fiber, so it helps with weight loss as well.

Cheese

Milk, as I will discuss in the next chapter, is not okay. You can get away with cheese though. Cheese is delicious and nutritious. Thankfully, although there are hundreds of types of cheese out there, all of them are low in carbs and full of fat. Eating cheese may even help your muscles and slow down aging.

Avocados

Avocados are so famous nowadays in the health community that people associate the word "health" to avocados. This is for a very good reason because avocados are very healthy. They pack lots of vitamins and minerals such as potassium. Moreover, avocados are shown to help the body go into ketosis faster.

Meat and Poultry

These two are the staple food in most keto diets. Most of the keto meals revolve around using these two ingredients. This is because they contain no carbs and pack plenty of vitamins and minerals. Moreover, they are a great source of protein.

Eggs

Eggs form the bulk of most food you will eat in a keto diet because they are the healthiest and most versatile food item of them all. Even a large egg contains so little carbs but packs plenty of protein, making it a perfect option for a keto diet.

Moreover, eggs are shown to have an appetite suppression effect, making you feel full for longer as well as regulating blood sugar levels. This leads to lower calorie intake for about a day. Just make sure to eat the entire egg because the nutrients are in the yolk.

Coconut Oil

Coconut oil and other coconut-related products such as coconut milk and coconut powder are perfect for a keto diet. Coconut oil, especially, contain MCTs that are converted into ketones by the liver to be used as an immediate source of energy.

Plain Greek Yogurt and Cottage Cheese

These two food items are rich in protein and a small number of carbs, small enough that you can safely include them into your keto diet. They also help suppress your appetite by making you feel full for longer and they can be eaten alone and are still delicious.

Olive Oil

Olive oil is very beneficial for your heart because it contains oleic acid that helps decrease heart disease risk factors. Extra-virgin olive oil is also rich in antioxidants. The best thing is that olive oil can be used as a main source of fat and it has no carbs. The same goes for olive.

Nuts and Seeds

These are also low in carbs but rich in fat. They are also healthy and have a lot of nutrients and fiber. They help reduce heart disease, cancer, depression, and other risks of diseases. The fiber in these also help make you feel full for longer, so you would consume fewer calories and your body would spend more calories digesting them.

Berries

Many fruits pack too many carbs that make them unsuitable in a keto diet, but not berries. They are low in carbs and high in fiber. Some of the best berries to include in your diet are blackberries, blueberries, raspberries, and strawberries.

Butter and Cream

These two food items pack plenty of fat and a very small amount of carbs, making them a good option to include in your keto diet.

Shirataki Noodles

If you love noodles and pasta but don't want to give up on them, then shirataki noodles are the perfect alternative. They are rich in water content and pack a lot of fiber, so that means low carbs and calories and hunger suppression.

Unsweetened Coffee and Tea

These two drinks are carb-free, so long as you don't add sugar, milk, or any other sweeteners. Both contain caffeine that improves your metabolism and suppresses your appetite. A word of warning to those who love light coffee and tea lattes, though. They are made with non-fat milk and contain a lot of carbs.

Dark Chocolate and Cocoa Powder

These two food items are delicious and contain antioxidants. Dark chocolate is associated with the reduction of heart disease risk by lowering the blood pressure. Just make sure that you choose only dark chocolate with at least 70% cocoa solids.

Foods to Avoid

In this chapter, I will show you the kinds of food you want to avoid at all costs. Because keto is a keto diet, that means you need to avoid high-carbs food. Some of the food you avoid is even healthy, but they just contain too many carbs. Here is a list of common food you should limit or avoid altogether.

Bread and Grains

Breads are a staple food in many countries. You have loaves, bagels, tortillas, the list goes on. However, no matter what form bread takes, they still pack a lot of carbs. The same applies to whole-grain as well because they are made from refined flour.

Depending on your daily carb limit, eating a sandwich or bagel can put you way over your daily limit. So if you really want to eat bread, it is best to make keto variants at home instead.

Grains such as rice, wheat, and oats pack a lot of carbs as well. So limit or avoid that as well.

Fruits

Fruits are healthy for you. In fact, they have been linked to a lower risk of heart disease and cancer. However, there are a few that you need to avoid in your keto diets. The problem is that some of those foods pack quite a lot of carbs such as banana, raisins, dates, mango, and pear.

As a general rule, avoid sweet and dried fruits. Berries are an exception because they do not contain as much sugar and are rich in fiber. So you can still eat some of them, around 50 grams. Moderation is key.

Vegetables

Vegetables are just as healthy for your body. Most of the keto diet does not care how many vegetables you eat so long as they are low in starch. Vegetables that are rich in fiber can help with weight loss. For one, they make you feel full for longer so they help suppress your appetite. Another benefit is that your body would burn more calories to break and digest them. Moreover, they help control blood sugar and aid with your bowel movements.

But that also means you need to avoid or limit vegetables that are high in starch because they have more carbs than fiber. That includes corn, potato, sweet potato, and beets.

Pasta

Pasta is also a staple food in many countries. It is versatile and convenient. As with any other convenient food, pasta is rich in carbs. So when you are on your keto diet, spaghetti or any other types of pasta are not recommended. You can probably get away with it by eating a small portion, but that is not possible.

Thankfully, that does not mean you need to give up on it altogether. If you are craving pasta, you can try some other alternatives that are low in carbs such as spiralized veggies or shirataki noodles.

Cereal

Cereal is also a huge offender because sugary breakfast cereals pack a lot of carbs. That also applies to "healthy cereals". Just because they use other words to describe their product does not mean that you should believe them. That also applies to oatmeal, whole-grain cereals, etc.

So when you eat a bowl of cereal when you are doing keto, you are already way over your carb limit, and we haven't even added milk into the equation! Therefore, avoid whole-grain cereal or cereals that we mention here altogether.

Beer

In reality, you can drink most alcoholic beverages in moderation without fear. For instance, dry wine does not have that many carbs and hard liquor has no carbs at all. So you can drink them without worry. Beer is an exception to this rule because it packs a lot of carbs.

Carbs in beers or other liquid are considered to be liquid carbs and they are even more dangerous than solid carbs. You see, when you eat food that is rich in carbs, you at least feel full. When you drink liquid carbs, you do not feel full as quickly so the appetite suppression effect is little.

Sweetened Yogurt

Yogurt is actually very healthy because it is tasty and does not have that many carbs. It is a very versatile food to have in your keto diet. The problem comes when you consume yogurt variants that are rich in carbs such as fruit-flavored, low-fat, sweetened, or nonfat yogurt. A single serving of sweetened yogurt actually contains as many carbs as a single serving of dessert.

If you really love yogurt, you can get away with half a cup of plain Greek yogurt with 50 grams of raspberries or blackberries.

Juice

Fruit juices are perhaps the worst beverage you can put into your system when you are on a keto diet. One may argue that juice provides some nutrients, but the problem is that it contains a lot of carbs that are very easy to digest. As a result, your blood sugar level will spike whenever you drink it. That also applies to vegetable juice because of the fast-digesting carbs present.

Another problem is that the brain does not process liquid carbs the same way as solid carbs. Solid carbs can help suppress appetite, but liquid carbs will only put your appetite into overdrive.

Low-fat and fat-free salad dressings

As mentioned previously, fruits and vegetables are largely okay so long as they are low in carbs. But if you have to buy salads, keep in mind that commercial dressings actually pack more carbs than you think, especially the fat-free and low-fat variants.

So if you want to enjoy your salad, dress your salad using creamy, full-fat dressing instead. To really cut down on carbs, you can use vinegar and olive oil, both of which are proven to help with heart health and aid in weight loss.

Beans and Legumes

These are also very nutritious as they are rich in fiber. Research has shown that eating these have many health benefits such as reduced inflammation and heart disease risk.

However, they are also rich in carbs. You may be able to enjoy a small amount of them when you are on your keto diet, but make sure you know exactly how much you can eat before you exceed your carb limit.

Sugar

We mean sugar in any form, including honey. You may already be aware of what foods that contain lots of sugar such as cookies, candies, and cake are forbidden on a keto diet or any other form of diet that is designed to lose weight.

What you may not be aware of is that nature's sugar such as honey is just as rich in carbs as processed sugar. In fact, natural forms of sugar contain even more carbs.

Not only that sugar, in general, is rich in carbs, they also add little to no nutritional value to your meal. When you are on a keto diet, you need to keep in mind that your diet is going to consist of food that is rich in fiber and nutritious. So sugar is out of the question.

If you really want to sweeten your food you can just use a healthy sweetener instead because they do not add as many carbs to your food.

Chips and Crackers

These two are some of the most popular snacks. What some people did not realize is that one packet of chips contain several servings and should not be all eaten in one go. The carbs can add up very quickly if you do not watch what you eat.

Crackers also pack a lot of carbs, although the amount varies based on how they are made. But even whole-wheat crackers contain a lot of carbs.

Due to how processed snacks are produced, it is difficult to stop yourself from eating everything within a short period of time. Therefore, it is advised that you avoid them altogether.

Milk

I mentioned previously that cereal contains a lot of carbs and a breakfast cereal will put you way over your carbs limit without you adding milk. Milk also contains a lot of carbs on its own. Therefore, avoid it if you can even though milk is a good source of many nutrients such as calcium, potassium, and other B vitamins.

Of course, that does not mean that you have to ditch milk altogether. You can get away with a tablespoon or two of milk for your coffee. But cream or half-and-half is better if you drink coffee frequently. These two contain very few carbs. But if you love to drink milk in large amounts or need it to make your favorite drinks, consider using coconut milk or unsweetened almond instead.

Gluten-free baked goods

Wheat, barley, and rye all contain gluten. Some people who have celiac disease still want to enjoy these delicacies but unable to because their gut will become inflamed in response to gluten. As such, gluten-free variants have been created to cater to their needs.

Gluten-free diets are very popular nowadays, but what many people don't seem to realize is that they pack quite a lot of carbs. That includes gluten-free bread, muffins, and other baked products. In reality, they contain even more carbs than their glutenous variant. Moreover, the flour used to make these gluten-free products are made from grains and starches. So when you consume a gluten-free bread, your blood sugar level spikes.

So, just stick to whole foods. Alternatively, you can use almond or coconut flour to make your own low-carb bread.

Tips on Losing Weight on Keto After 50

In this chapter, I will go over a few more things you can do so you can optimize your weight loss.

Exercise

In the fitness world, it is already established that 80% of your weight loss success comes from the diet. So just by following the keto diet alone, you are already making great progress. However, if you want that extra edge in your weight loss, consider doing exercises.

You have plenty of options here. You can do cardio exercises such as jogging, running or cycling every morning for 30 minutes, but strength training works just as well for older adults. In fact, you should do both if you can.

Cardio exercises can get the heart pumping and get the body moving more freely, but note that your muscle mass starts to decline after 50. So work on your muscles as well.

How much exercise should you do? It depends on how much you can handle. No point in pushing beyond the limit and regret it later, right?

Team Up

A group activity is always more entertaining. So if you can find like-minded individuals who are also into keto diets, consider doing it together with them. It makes things much easier. This tip also applies to some other tips that I will show you, such as exercise that I just covered.

Move More

Moving more here does not mean more cardio exercises. You cannot expect to get any more effective weight loss if you exercise for 30mns a day and then sit on the couch for the rest of the day. The idea is to burn more calories than you can take in, so it pays to be a little extra active throughout the day.

If you have a desk job, consider getting up at least once an hour and take a short break by walking in the lobby for at least 5 minutes. It doesn't seem much, but it helps in the long run.

More Protein

Protein is very important for both weight loss and youth, including the protection against muscle degradation and other aging ailments. Couple a high protein intake with strength exercise and you can be sure that you would be building muscles faster than they can degrade. You won't look like Arnold when he was a bodybuilder, but you might even look fitter than the guy in his 20s at your workplace.

Talk to a Dietitian

The first thing you should do before getting into any diet is to consult your dietitian. While the keto diet works for many people, you never really know if it will work for you. Therefore, it is wise to ask your dietitian first before you jump in, rather than suffer some adverse effects because your body is not compatible with this diet.

Cook at Home More

Or eat out less frequently. There are two reasons why you should do that. For one, there are only a few places, if at all, that serve keto-based foods, let alone those that follow your diet plan. You need to prepare your own food if you want to do a keto diet. Another benefit is economics. You will buy most of your ingredients and prepare your meals ahead of time. This means you will only spend your money on the ingredients you know you will need.

Eat More Produce

While we are on the subject of eating, consider incorporating more produces in your diet, some of which I have covered already. Vegetables and fruits are full of nutrients that your body needs to remain healthy, so it should be included in your diet.

Hire a Personal Trainer

While we are still discussing exercising, consider getting yourself a personal trainer. That way, you can get the most out of your exercises and your trainer also doubles as an exercise partner as well because they hold you accountable for your own commitments. Your trainer is very helpful when you do strength training because they can teach you how to perform the exercise with the correct form and preventing you from injuring yourself.

Rely Less on Convenience Foods

Convenient foods are convenient, but not healthy. Not by a long shot. They are rich in calories and often do not pack essential nutrients such as protein, fiber, vitamins, etc. If you can, ditch convenient foods altogether.

Find an Activity You Enjoy

When you have done enough exercise, you will know what activities you like. One way to encourage yourself to exercise more regularly is by making it entertaining than a chore. If possible, stick to your favorite activities and you can get the most out of your exercises. Keep in mind that the activities you enjoy may not be effective or needed, so you need to find other exercises to compensate, which you may not enjoy so much. For instance, if you like jogging, then you can really work your leg muscles, but your arms are not involved. So you need to do pushups or other strength training exercises.

Here, your trainer can help you decide and create a workout routine that you can stick with as well.

Check with a Healthcare Provider

As mentioned earlier, the keto diet works for many people, but it isn't for everyone. Your dietitian can tell you whether keto diet would work, but it helps to check in with your healthcare provider to ensure that you do not have any medical condition that prevents you from losing weight, such as hypothyroidism and polycystic ovarian syndrome. It helps to know well in advance whether your body is even capable of losing fat in the first place before you commit and see no result, right?

Eat Less at Night

While the science still argues about it to this day, it seems more logical that breakfast is the most important meal of the day considering that you would not have eaten for the past 8 hours whereas the interval between breakfast and lunch, and lunch and dinner is 5 or 6 hours at best. By the same token, dinner should be small because your body does not need to expend that much energy when you are sleeping anyway. So the excess energy becomes fat.

So keep dinner light. For one, it helps you lose weight. Another reason is if you have a heavy dinner, your body will strain itself trying to digest everything. That means your body would remain active until all the food is digested, meaning that you will not get restful sleep if you can sleep at all.

Bottom line: Eat light and eat dinner at least 4 hours prior to bedtime. Any sooner and you will have a hard time sleeping.

Body Composition

Your body isn't just "weight" alone. Your body is composed of fat, muscles, fluid, bones, etc. What you want to lose is fat weight, not muscle weight or fluid weight. You want as little fat mass in your body as possible while still maintaining a healthy level of non-fat mass in your body. There are many ways you can measure your body fat, but the simplest method is to measure your calves, thighs, waist, chest, and biceps.

Hydrate Properly

That means drinking enough water or herbal tea and ditch sweetened beverages or other drinks that contain sugar altogether. Making the transition will be difficult for the first few weeks, but your body will be thanking you for it. There is nothing healthier than good old plain water and the recommended amount is 2 gallons a day. However, because you are on a keto diet, your body needs to use up more water so consider 2 gallons to the absolute minimum amount of water you need to drinks. I recommend you drink between 3 or even 4 gallons a day when you are on a keto diet. If you get thirsty, then it is a sign of dehydration, so drink some water. Drinking plenty of water also leads to additional calories burned. You can shave off a few more calories by drinking cold water because your body will spend more energy trying to regulate your body temperature.

Supplements

When you get older, your body starts to lose its ability to absorb certain nutrients, which leads to deficits. For example, vitamin B12 and folate are some of the most common nutrients that people over 50 lack. They have an impact on your mood, energy level, and weight loss rate.

Therefore, if you feel tired when you are on your keto diet, perhaps you do not get enough nutrients that your body needs. That does not mean you should eat more, no. You just need to take the right supplements.

Get Enough Sleep

When you are over 50, your body starts to fail you. You no longer have the ability to party past midnight without feeling horrible for the rest of the month. If there is the most crucial time to get 8 hours of sleep a day, then it is right now.

Getting enough sleep helps your body regulate the hormones in your body, so try to aim for 7 to 9 hours of sleep a day. You can get more restful sleep by creating a nighttime routine that involves not looking at a computer, phone, or TV screen for at least 1 hour before bed. You can drink warm milk or water to help your body relax, or even do 10 to 20 minutes of stretching so you can get a restful sleep.

While we are on the subject of sleeping, try to maintain a consistent sleeping schedule. I understand that you want to sleep and wake up 1 to 4 hours later than usual during the weekend. But you want to go to bed and wake up at the same time, your mood and energy level will be higher. An added benefit is that your body will learn to wake up on its own even without the alarm.

Mindful Eating

Mindfulness isn't restricted to meditation alone. Again, we will not go over meditation in this book because it is another topic altogether. But what you can do here is learn to love and appreciate your food. It sounds obnoxious, but it helps your mood and promotes weight loss.

Simply put, you just have to put away your phone and take away any other sources of distractions and focus solely on your food, how it tastes, etc. That means eating slowly. You will learn to appreciate how tasty your food is because you actually focus on eating.

How does this translate to weight loss? You see, there is a system in your body that determines how full you are. The issue here is that this system is not instantaneous. It takes some time to measure how full your stomach it before sending the signal to your brain. So when you eat too quickly, by the time you feel full, you would have already overshot by a country mile. If you eat slowly, your body has enough time to register your fullness bite by bite. So when you feel full, you have not overeaten.

Use Inconvenience to Your Advantage

In the last chapter, I pointed out that eating chips, crackers, or any other salty snacks can cause you to overeat very quickly. The problem is that just ditching these delicious snacks cold turkey style is difficult, especially if you have developed a taste for them. So what do you do? Well, you remove such food from your house immediately. Only have enough food in the house for the week or have only healthy snacks in the house.

Even when you have a sudden craving for unhealthy snacks, the inconvenience of going out to buy one is enough to dissuade you and help you suppress the hunger. Another solution is to tell yourself that you will grab that unhealthy snack "tomorrow". We are all professional procrastinators or were one at a certain point in our lives, so use that to your advantage as well. When you set a "plan" like that, your mind is tricked into thinking that you will get around to it when the time is right, although that time will never come.

But what if you need to go out and get groceries for next week's keto meals? You have two options.

You can go to the grocery store carrying just enough money to get everything you need for next week's meals. That way, you simply cannot afford to buy extra snacks. But this requires your prior knowledge of the prices of the products you need to buy, and any price changes can leave you with some extra change or you not having enough money. To remedy this problem, I recommend you bring a bit extra just in case there are any price changes.

An alternative that I like is to bring someone along with you for the trip, but you let them carry all the money. The amount does not matter here, but it requires the other person to be firm about not letting you buy that potato chip. They have the money and they will have to stick to the plan of buying enough for the week, nothing more than that. It is going to be a bit inconvenient for the other person, but they can hold you accountable and keep you in control of the situation.

21-Day Keto Meal Plan for People Over 50

In this chapter, I will give you a 21-day keto meal plan so you know exactly what you need to eat for each day.

	Breakfast	Lunch	Dinner	Nutritional Values
Day 1	Avocado Bun Breakfast Burger	Avocado Cream and Zoodles	Chicken Cutlet and Cauli Rice	Calories: 1765 Fat: 139.05g Protein:90.91g Net carbs: 20.75g
Day 2	Breakfast Sausage, Eggs & Greens	Chicken Cutlet & Cauli Rice	Shirataki Noodles Asian Salad	Calories: 1374 Fat: 93g Protein: 98.61g Net Carbs: 19.79g
Day 3	Breakfast Sausage & Eggs	BLT Lettuce Boats	Grilled Cod & Shrimps	Calories: 1177 Fat: 78.94g Protein: 94.65g Net Carbs: 15.74g
Day 4	90-sec Sausage Egg Muffin	Grilled Cod & Shrimps	Arugula Caesar Salad & Veggies	Calories: 1316 Fat: 89g Net Carbs: 19.75g Protein: 99.06g
Day 5	Breakfast Sausage & Poached Egg	Rosemary Chicken & Broccoli	Rosemary Pork Roast Side Caesar Salad	Calories: 1495 Fat: 111.31g Net Carbs: 12.34g Protein: 101.2g
Day 6	Spinach & Breakfast Sausage	Rosemary Pork Roast Side Caesar	Broccoli, Bacon & Mushrooms	Calories: 1313 Fat: 99.55g Protein: 84.98g

	Omelet	Salad 2		Net carbs: 13.02g
Day 7	Spinach & Pork Omelet	Zucchini Salad with Grilled Chicken Thigh	Rosemary Pork Roast Side Caesar Salad	Calories: 1509 Fat: 114.98g Protein: 96.37g Net carbs: 15.62g
Day 8	Chorizo Breakfast Bake	Sesame Pork Lettuce Wraps	Avocado Lime Salmon	Calories: 1,520 Fat: 109g Protein: 110g Net Carbs: 16g
Day 9	Chorizo Breakfast Bake with 3 Slices Thick-Cut Bacon	Spiced Pumpkin Soup	Avocado Lime Salmon	Calories: 1,570 Fat: 124g Protein: 92g Net Carbs: 16
Day 10	Baked Eggs in Avocado	Easy Beef Curry	Easy Beef Curry	Calories: 1,700 Fat: 128.5g Protein: 103g Net Carbs: 22g
Day 11	Lemon Poppy Ricotta Pancakes with 3 Slices Thick-Cut Bacon	Spiced Pumpkin Soup with ½ Medium Avocado	Rosemary Roasted Chicken and Veggies	Calories: 1,665 Fat: 130g Protein: 95.5g Net Carbs: 23.5g
Day 12	Lemon Poppy Ricotta Pancakes	Spiced Pumpkin Soup	Cheesy Sausage Mushroom Skillet with	Calories: 1,650 Fat: 126g Protein: 100.5g Net Carbs: 22.5g

			1 Slice Thick-Cut Bacon	
Day 13	Sweet Blueberry Coconut Porridge with 1 Slice Thick-Cut Bacon	Easy Beef Curry	Cheesy Sausage Mushroom Skillet	Calories: 1,670 Fat: 112g Protein: 100g Net Carbs: 33.5g
Day 14	Sweet Blueberry Coconut Porridge	Easy Beef Curry	Lamb Chops with Rosemary and Garlic	Calories: 1,625 Fat: 108g Protein: 110.5g Net Carbs: 27g
Day 15	Pepper Jack Sausage Egg Muffins with ½ Medium Avocado	Cabbage and Sausage Skillet with 1 Slice Thick-Cut Bacon	Gyro Salad with Avo-Tzatziki	Calories: 1,605 Fat: 118.5g Protein: 102g Net Carbs: 22.5g
Day 16	Fat-Busting Vanilla Protein Smoothie	Easy Cheeseburger Salad	Chicken Zoodle Alfredo	Calories: 1,530 Fat: 113.5g Protein: 107.5g Net Carbs: 18.5g
Day 17	Pepper Jack Sausage Egg Muffins with 1 Slice Thick-Cut Bacon	Pan-Fried Pepperoni Pizza	Gyro Salad with Avo-Tzatziki	Calories: 1,650 Fat: 127.5g Protein: 101g Net Carbs: 29g

Day				
Day 18	Savory Ham and Cheese Waffles with 2 Slices Thick-Cut Bacon	Pan-Fried Pepperoni Pizzas	Cabbage and Sausage Skillet	Calories: 1,670 Fat: 129g Protein: 103g Net Carbs: 20.5g
Day 19	Savory Ham and Cheese Waffles with 1 Slice Thick-Cut Bacon	Cabbage and Sausage Skillet	Chicken Zoodle Alfredo	Calories: 1,620 Fat: 119g Protein: 119g Net Carbs: 18.5g
Day 20	Mozzarella Veggie-Loaded Quiche with 1 Slice Thick-Cut Bacon	Easy Cheeseburger Salad	Gyro Salad with Avo-Tzatziki	Calories: 1,580 Fat: 104.5g Protein: 117.5g Net Carbs: 33g
Day 21	Pepper Jack Sausage Egg Muffins with 3 Slices Thick-Cut Bacon	Pan-Fried Pepperoni Pizza	Cabbage and Sausage Skillet	Calories: 1,650 Fat: 127.5g Protein: 101g Net Carbs: 29g

Keep in mind that this meal plan is not for everyone because of allergies or other medical complications, so at least consult your doctor and see what food you cannot eat and customize accordingly. So long as you know how much carbs, fat, and protein you need to consume, you are good to go.

Breakfast Recipes

Kale Wrapped Eggs

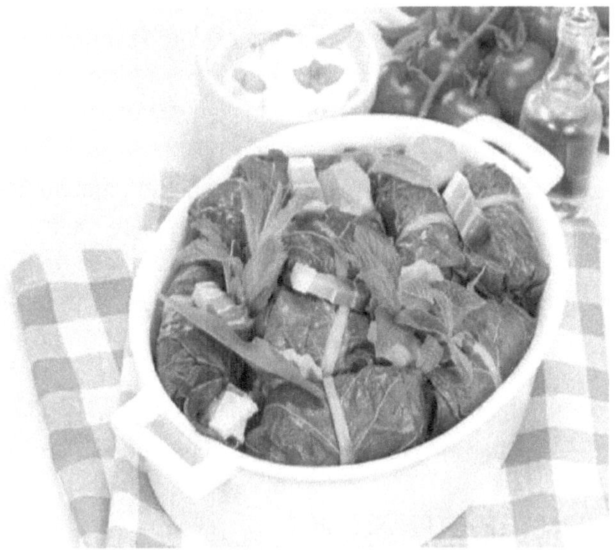

Prep Time: 8-10 min.

Cooking Time: 5 min.

Number of Servings: 4

Ingredients:

- Three tablespoons heavy cream
- Four hardboiled eggs
- ¼ teaspoon pepper
- Four kale leaves
- Four prosciutto slices
- ¼ teaspoon salt
- 1 ½ cups water

Directions:

1. Peel the eggs and wrap each with the kale. Wrap them in the
   prosciutto slices and sprinkle with ground black pepper and

salt.

2. Arrange Instant Pot over a dry platform in your kitchen. Open its top lid and switch it on.
3. In the pot, pour water. Arrange a trivet or steamer basket inside that came with Instant Pot. Now place/arrange the eggs over the trivet/basket.
4. Close the lid to create a locked chamber; make sure that safety valve is in locking position.
5. Find and press "MANUAL" cooking function; timer to 5 minutes with default "HIGH" pressure mode.
6. Allow the pressure to build to cook the ingredients.
7. After cooking time is over press "CANCEL" setting. Find and press "QPR" cooking function. This setting is for quick release of inside pressure.
8. Slowly open the lid, take out the cooked recipe in serving plates or serving bowls, and enjoy the keto recipe.

Nutritional Values (Per Serving):

Calories - 247

Fat – 20g

Saturated Fat – 6g

Trans Fat – 0g

Carbohydrates – 7g

Fiber – 3g

Sodium – 742mg

Protein – 19g

Zucchini Keto Bread

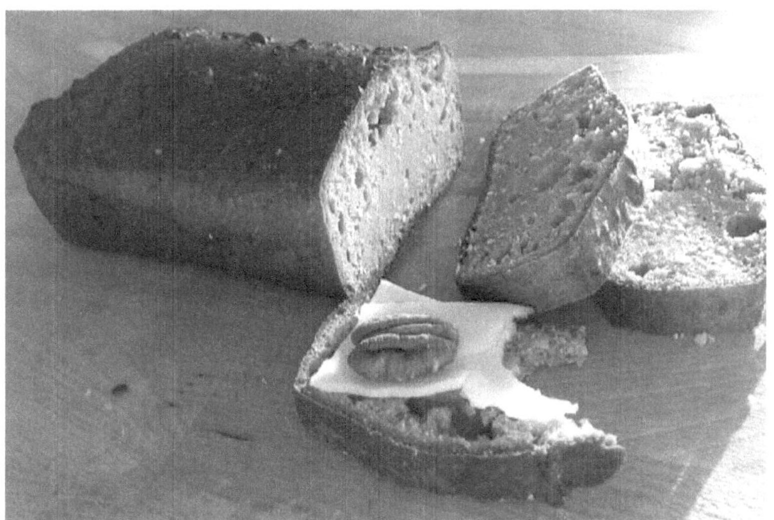

Prep Time: 8-10 min.

Cooking Time: 40 min.

Number of Servings: 12-16 slices

Ingredients:

- 1 cup grated zucchini
- 2 ½ cups almond flour
- ½ cup chopped walnuts
- 3 eggs
- ½ cup olive oil
- 1 ½ teaspoon baking powder
- Pinch of ginger powder
- 1 teaspoon vanilla extract
- ½ teaspoon cinnamon
- ¼ teaspoon nutmeg
- pinch of sea salt
- 1 ½ cups water

Directions:

1. Whisk together the wet ingredients in a bowl.
2. Combine the dry ingredients in another bowl. Combine the dry and wet mixture. Stir in the zucchini.
3. Grease a loaf pan with some butter and pour the mixture. Top with chopped walnuts.
4. Arrange Instant Pot over a dry platform in your kitchen. Open its top lid and switch it on.
5. In the pot, pour water. Arrange a trivet or steamer basket inside that came with Instant Pot. Now place/arrange the loaf pan over the trivet/basket.
6. Close the lid to create a locked chamber; make sure that safety valve is in locking position.
7. Find and press "MANUAL" cooking function; timer to 40 minutes with default "HIGH" pressure mode.
8. Allow the pressure to build to cook the ingredients.
9. After cooking time is over press "CANCEL" setting. Find and press "QPR" cooking function. This setting is for quick release of inside pressure.
10. Slowly open the lid, take out the cooked bread.
11. Cooldown, slice, and serve.

Nutritional Values (Per Serving):

Calories – 164

Fat – 17g

Saturated Fat – 2g

Trans Fat – 0g

Carbohydrates – 3g

Fiber – 2g

Sodium – 94mg

Protein – 5g

Ham Sausage Quiche

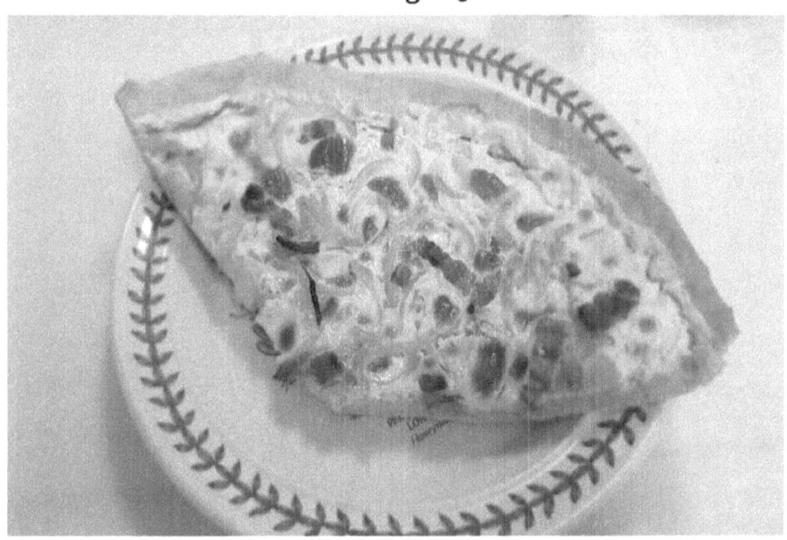

Prep Time: 8-10 min.

Cooking Time: 30 min.

Number of Servings: 4

Ingredients:

- 4 bacon slices, cooked and crumbled
- ½ cup diced ham
- 2 green onions, chopped
- ½ cup full-fat milk
- Six eggs, beaten
- 1 cup ground sausage, cooked
- 1 cup shredded cheddar cheese
- ¼ teaspoon salt
- Pinch of pepper
- 1 ½ cups water

Directions:

1. Grease a baking dish with coconut oil cooking spray.
2. Place all of the ingredients in a bowl, and stir to combine. Add

this mixture to the prepared dish.

3. Arrange Instant Pot over a dry platform in your kitchen. Open its top lid and switch it on.
4. In the pot, pour water. Arrange a trivet or steamer basket inside that came with Instant Pot. Now place/arrange the dish over the trivet/basket.
5. Close the lid to create a locked chamber; make sure that safety valve is in locking position.
6. Find and press "MANUAL" cooking function; timer to 30 minutes with default "HIGH" pressure mode.
7. Allow the pressure to build to cook the ingredients.
8. After cooking time is over press "CANCEL" setting. Find and press "QPR" cooking function. This setting is for quick release of inside pressure.

9. Place the dish on the rack in your IP and close the lid. Cook on HIGH for 30 minutes release the pressure naturally, for 10 minutes.
10. Slowly open the lid, take out the cooked recipe in serving plates or serving bowls, and enjoy the keto recipe.

Nutritional Values (Per Serving):

Calories - 398

Fat – 31g

Saturated Fat – 13g

Trans Fat – 0g

Carbohydrates – 5g

Fiber – 1g

Sodium – 745mg

Protein – 26g

Coconut Almond Breakfast

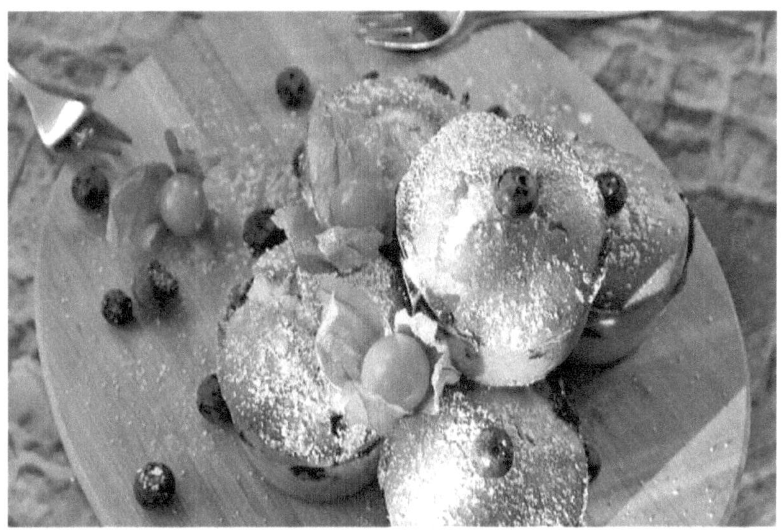

Prep Time: 8-10 min.

Cooking Time: 5 min.

Number of Servings: 2

Ingredients:

- 2 tablespoons roasted pepitas
- 1/3 cup coconut milk
- 2 tablespoon chopped almonds
- 1 tablespoon chia seeds
- 1/3 cup water
- One handful blueberries

Directions:

1. In your food processor or blender, mix the pepitas with almonds and pulse them well.
2. Arrange Instant Pot over a dry platform in your kitchen. Open its top lid and switch it on.
3. Add the chia seeds with water and coconut milk; gently stir to mix well.

4. Add the pepita mix and combine.
5. Close the lid to create a locked chamber; make sure that safety valve is in locking position.
6. Find and press "MANUAL" cooking function; timer to 5 minutes with default "HIGH" pressure mode.
7. Allow the pressure to build to cook the ingredients.
8. After cooking time is over press "CANCEL" setting. Find and press "QPR" cooking function. This setting is for quick release of inside pressure.
9. Slowly open the lid, take out the cooked recipe in serving plates or serving bowls, top with the blueberries, and enjoy the keto recipe.

Nutritional Values (Per Serving):

Calories - 148

Fat – 6g

Saturated Fat – 1g

Trans Fat – 0g

Carbohydrates – 4g

Fiber – 1.5g

Sodium – 346mg

Protein – 2g

Avocado Egg Muffins

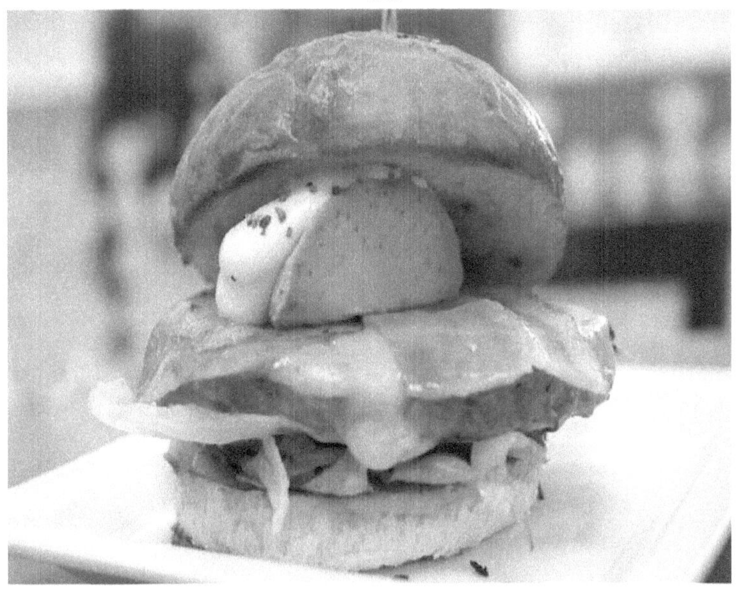

Prep Time: 8-10 min.

Cooking Time: 12 min.

Number of Servings: 4

Ingredients:

- 1 ½ cups of coconut milk
- 2 avocados, diced
- 4 ½ ounces (grated or shredded) cheese
- ½ cup almond flour
- 5 bacon slices, cooked and crumbled
- 5 eggs, beaten
- 2 tablespoon butter
- 3 spring onions, diced
- 1 teaspoon oregano
- ¼ cup flaxseed meal
- 1 ½ tablespoon lemon juice
- 1 teaspoon minced garlic
- 1 teaspoon onion powder

- 1 teaspoon salt
- Pinch of pepper
- 1 teaspoon baking powder
- 1 ½ cups water

Directions:

1. Whisk together the wet ingredients.
2. Gradually stir in the dry ingredients; mix until turns smooth. Stir in the avocado, bacon, onions, and cheese.
3. Add the mixture into 16 muffin cups.
4. Arrange Instant Pot over a dry platform in your kitchen. Open its top lid and switch it on.
5. In the pot, pour water. Arrange a trivet or steamer basket inside that came with Instant Pot. Now place/arrange the 8 cups over the trivet/basket.
6. Close the lid to create a locked chamber; make sure that safety valve is in locking position.
7. Find and press "MANUAL" cooking function; timer to 12 minutes with default "HIGH" pressure mode.
8. Allow the pressure to build to cook the ingredients.
9. After cooking time is over press "CANCEL" setting. Find and press "QPR" cooking function. This setting is for quick release of inside pressure.
10. Slowly open the lid, take out the cooked recipe in serving plates or serving bowls, and enjoy the keto recipe.
11. Repeat the same process.

Nutritional Values (Per Serving):

Calories - 146

Fat – 11g

Saturated Fat – 3g

Trans Fat – 0g

Carbohydrates – 4g

Fiber – 2g

Sodium – 356mg

Protein – 6g

Lunch

Super Herbed Fish

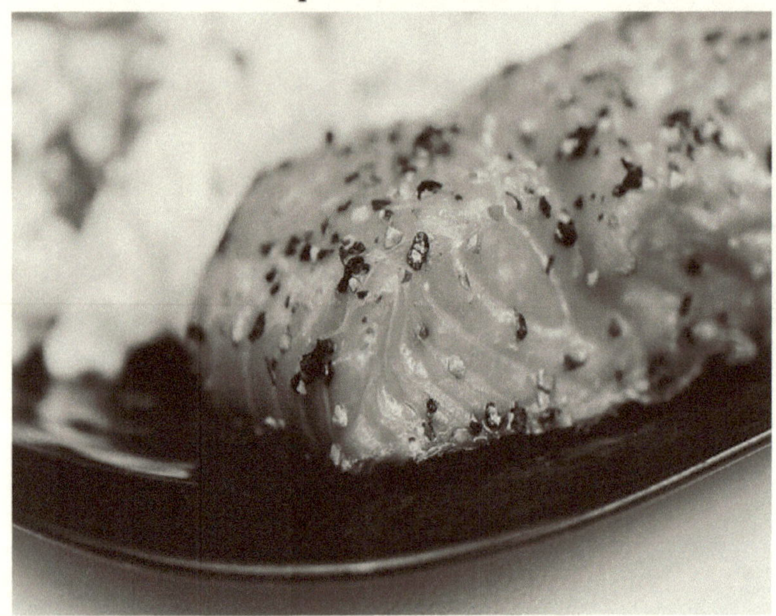

Prep Time: 8-10 min.

Cooking Time: 6 min.

Number of Servings: 1

Ingredients:

- 1 tablespoon chopped basil
- 2 teaspoons lime zest
- 1 tablespoon lime juice
- 1 tablespoon olive oil
- 1 4-ounce fish fillet
- 1 rosemary sprig
- 1 thyme sprig
- 1 teaspoon Dijon mustard
- ¼ teaspoon garlic powder
- Pinch of salt

- Pinch of pepper
- 1 ½ cups water

Directions:

1. Season the fish with salt and paper. Arrange on a piece of parchment paper and sprinkle with zest.
2. Whisk together the oil, juice, and mustard in a mixing bowl and brush over. Top with the herbs.
3. Wrap the fish with the parchment paper. Wrap the wrapped fish in an aluminum foil.
4. Arrange Instant Pot over a dry platform in your kitchen. Open its top lid and switch it on.
5. In the pot, pour water. Arrange a trivet or steamer basket inside that came with Instant Pot. Now place/arrange the foil over the trivet/basket.
6. Close the lid to create a locked chamber; make sure that safety valve is in locking position.
7. Find and press "MANUAL" cooking function; timer to 5 minutes with default "HIGH" pressure mode.
8. Allow the pressure to build to cook the ingredients.
9. After cooking time is over press "CANCEL" setting. Find and press "QPR" cooking function. This setting is for quick release of inside pressure.
10. Slowly open the lid, take out the cooked recipe in serving plates or serving bowls, and enjoy the keto recipe.

Nutritional Values (Per Serving):

Calories - 246

Fat – 9g

Saturated Fat – 1g

Trans Fat – 0g

Carbohydrates – 1g

Fiber – 0.5g

Sodium – 86mg

Protein – 28g

Turkey Avocado Chili

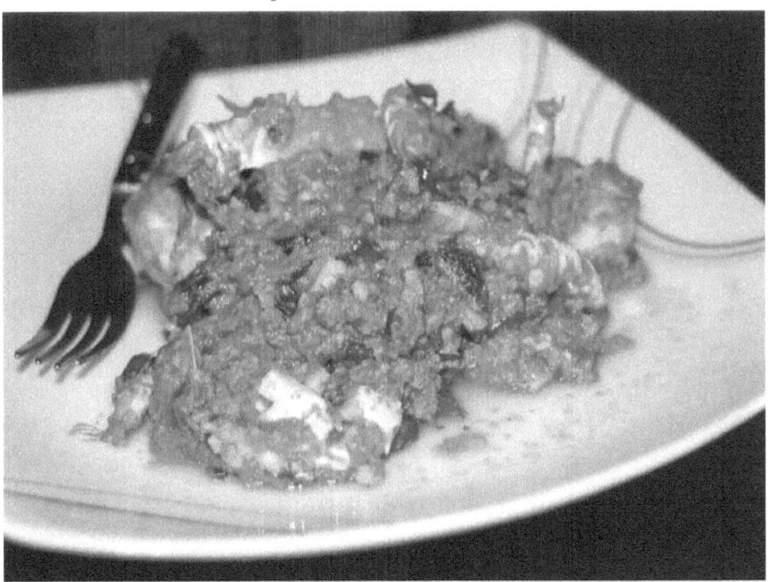

Prep Time: 8-10 min.

Cooking Time: 50 min.

Number of Servings: 3-4

Ingredients:

- 2 ½ pounds lean (finely ground) turkey
- 2 cups diced tomatoes
- 2-ounce tomato paste, sugar-free
- 1 tablespoon olive oil
- ½ chopped large yellow onion
- 8 minced garlic cloves
- 1 (4-ounce) can green chilies with liquid
- 2 tablespoons Worcestershire sauce
- 1 tablespoon dried oregano
- ¼ cup red chili powder
- 2 tablespoons (finely ground) cumin
- Salt and freshly (finely ground) black pepper, as per taste preference
- 1 pitted and sliced avocado, peeled

Directions:

1. Arrange Instant Pot over a dry platform in your kitchen. Open its top lid and switch it on.
2. Find and press "SAUTE" cooking function; add the oil in it and allow it to heat.
3. In the pot, add the onions; cook (while stirring) until turns translucent and softened for around 4-5 minutes.
4. Add the garlic and cook for about 1 minute.
5. Add the turkey and cook for about 8-9 minutes. Stir in remaining ingredients except for the avocado.
6. Close the lid to create a locked chamber; make sure that safety valve is in locking position.
7. Find and press "MEAT/STEW" cooking function; timer to 35 minutes with default "HIGH" pressure mode.
8. Allow the pressure to build to cook the ingredients.
9. After cooking time is over press "CANCEL" setting. Find and press "NPR" cooking function. This setting is for the natural release of inside pressure, and it takes around 10 minutes to release pressure slowly.
10. Slowly open the lid, take out the cooked recipe in serving plates or serving bowls, top with the avocado slices, and enjoy the keto recipe.

Nutritional Values (Per Serving):

Calories - 346

Fat – 19g

Saturated Fat – 4g

Trans Fat – 0g

Carbohydrates – 7g

Fiber – 5g

Sodium – 246mg

Protein – 29g

Cheesy Tomato Shrimp

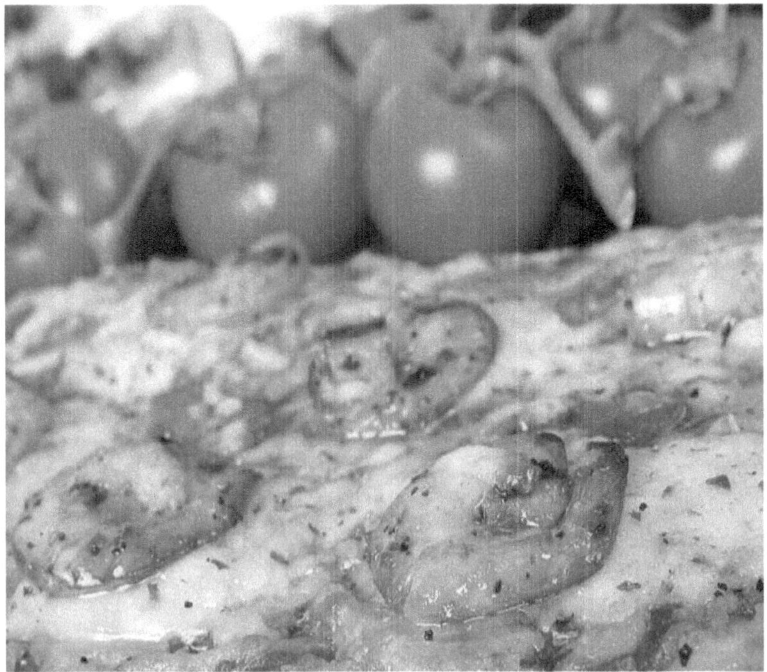

Prep Time: 8-10 min.

Cooking Time: 15 min.

Number of Servings: 4

Ingredients:

- 2 tablespoons olive oil
- ½ cup veggie broth
- ¼ cup chopped cilantro
- 2 tablespoons lime juice
- 1 ½ pounds shrimp, peeled and deveined
- 1 ½ pounds tomatoes, chopped
- 1 jalapeno, diced
- 1 onion, diced
- 1 cup shredded cheddar cheese
- 1 teaspoon minced garlic

Directions:

1. Arrange Instant Pot over a dry platform in your kitchen. Open its top lid and switch it on.
2. Find and press "SAUTE" cooking function; add the oil in it and allow it to heat.
3. In the pot, add the onions; cook (while stirring) until turns translucent and softened for around 2-3 minutes.
4. Add garlic and sauté for 30-60 seconds.
5. Stir in the broth, cilantro, and tomatoes.
6. Close the lid to create a locked chamber; make sure that safety valve is in locking position.
7. Find and press "MANUAL" cooking function; timer to 9 minutes with default "HIGH" pressure mode.
8. Allow the pressure to build to cook the ingredients.
9. After cooking time is over press "CANCEL" setting. Find and press "NPR" cooking function. This setting is for the natural release of inside pressure, and it takes around 10 minutes to release pressure slowly.
10. Add the shrimps.
11. Close the top lid to create a locked chamber; make sure that safety valve is in locking position.
12. Find and press "MANUAL" cooking function; timer to 2 minutes with default "HIGH" pressure mode.
13. Allow the pressure to build to cook the ingredients.
14. After cooking time is over press "CANCEL" setting. Find and press "NPR" cooking function. This setting is for the natural release of inside pressure, and it takes around 10 minutes to release pressure slowly.
15. Slowly open the lid, take out the cooked recipe in serving plates or serving bowls, top with the cheddar, and enjoy the keto recipe.

Nutritional Values (Per Serving):

Calories - 268

Fat – 16g

Saturated Fat – 5g

Trans Fat – 0g

Carbohydrates – 7g

Fiber – 2g

Sodium – 208mg

Protein – 22g

Cajun Rosemary Chicken

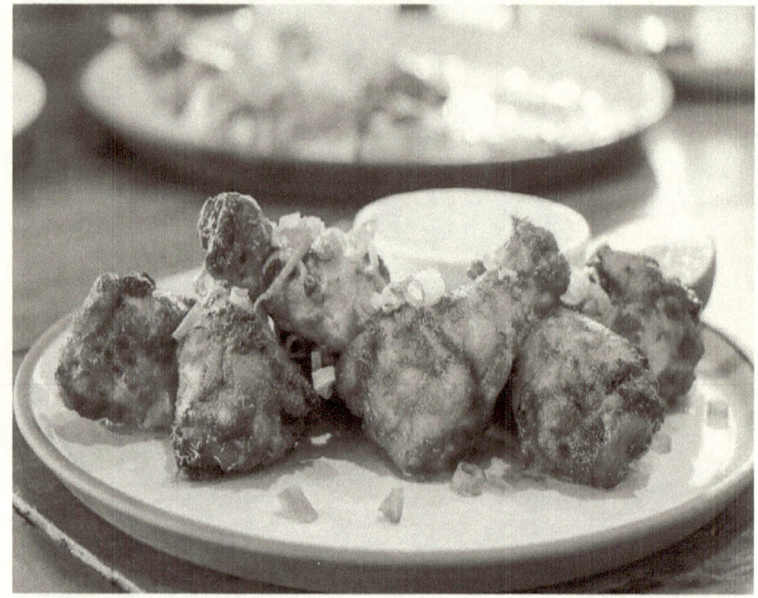

Prep Time: 8-10 min.

Cooking Time: 30 min.

Number of Servings: 4

Ingredients:

- 2 teaspoons Cajun seasoning
- 1 lemon, halved
- 1 yellow onion, make quarters
- 1 teaspoon garlic salt
- 1 medium chicken
- 2 rosemary sprigs
- 1 tablespoon coconut oil
- 1/4 teaspoon pepper
- 1 1/2 cups chicken broth

Directions:

1. Season the chicken with garlic salt, pepper, and Cajun

seasoning. Stuff the lemon, onion, and rosemary in the chicken's cavity.
2. Arrange Instant Pot over a dry platform in your kitchen. Open its top lid and switch it on.
3. Find and press "SAUTE" cooking function; add the oil in it and allow it to heat.
4. In the pot, add the meat; cook (while stirring) until turns evenly brown from all sides.
5. Add the broth; gently stir to mix well.
6. Close the lid to create a locked chamber; make sure that safety valve is in locking position.
7. Find and press "MANUAL" cooking function; timer to 25 minutes with default "HIGH" pressure mode.
8. Allow the pressure to build to cook the ingredients.
9. After cooking time is over press "CANCEL" setting. Find and press "NPR" cooking function. This setting is for the natural release of inside pressure, and it takes around 10 minutes to release pressure slowly.
10. Slowly open the lid, take out the cooked recipe in serving plates or serving bowls, and enjoy the keto recipe.

Nutritional Values (Per Serving):

Calories - 236

Fat – 26g

Saturated Fat – 7g

Trans Fat – 0g

Carbohydrates – 1g

Fiber – 5g

Sodium – 426mg

Protein – 31g

Chicken Spinach Curry

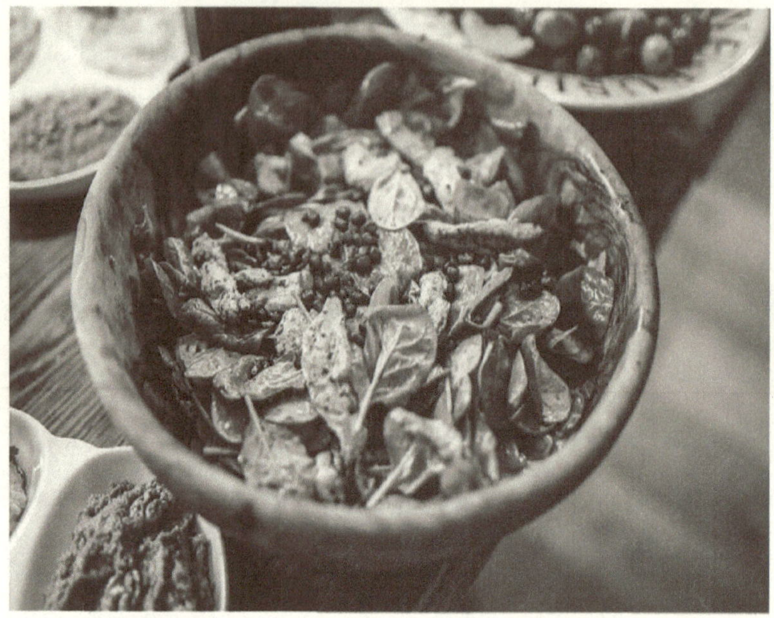

Prep Time: 8-10 min.

Cooking Time: 17 min.

Number of Servings: 3-4

Ingredients:

- 2 tomatoes, chopped
- 4 ounces spinach, chopped
- 1/3 pound curry paste
- 1 1/2 cups yogurt
- 4 pounds chicken, cubed
- 1 tablespoon olive oil
- 1 onion, cut to make slices
- 1 tablespoon chopped coriander

Directions:

1. Combine the chicken, curry paste, and yogurt in a mixing bowl. Cover and marinate in the fridge for 30 minutes.

2. Arrange Instant Pot over a dry platform in your kitchen. Open its top lid and switch it on.
3. Find and press "SAUTE" cooking function; add the oil in it and allow it to heat.
4. In the pot, add the onions; cook (while stirring) until turns translucent and softened.
5. Add the tomatoes and cook for another minute.
6. Pour the chicken mixture, mix in the spinach and coriander; gently stir to mix well.
7. Close the lid to create a locked chamber; make sure that safety valve is in locking position.
8. Find and press "MANUAL" cooking function; timer to 15 minutes with default "HIGH" pressure mode.
9. Allow the pressure to build to cook the ingredients.
10. After cooking time is over press "CANCEL" setting. Find and press "QPR" cooking function. This setting is for quick release of inside pressure.
11. Slowly open the lid, take out the cooked recipe in serving plates or serving bowls, and enjoy the keto recipe.

Nutritional Values (Per Serving):

Calories - 384

Fat – 18g

Saturated Fat – 3g

Trans Fat – 0g

Carbohydrates – 12g

Fiber – 6g

Sodium – 182mg

Protein – 39g

Dinner

Sriracha Tuna Kabobs

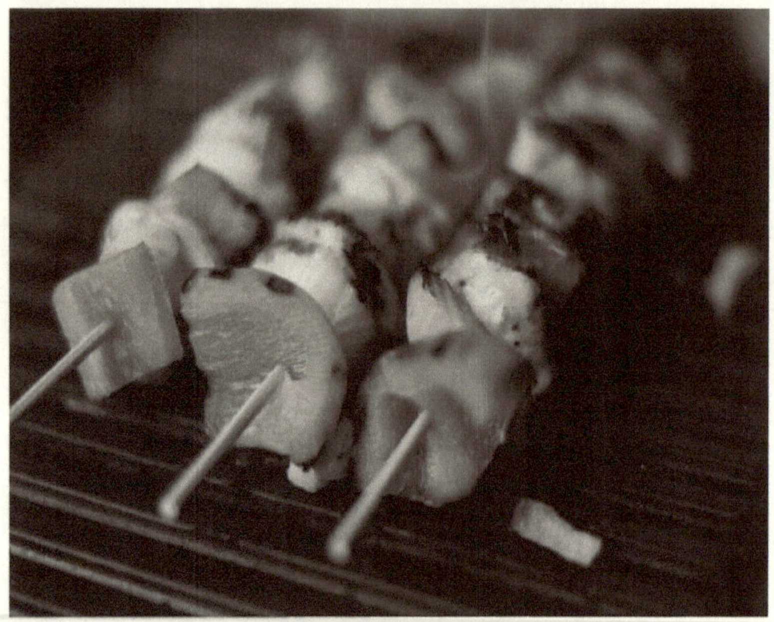

Prep time: 4 minutes

Cook time: 9 minutes

Number of Servings: 4

Ingredients

- 4 tablespoon Huy Fong chili garlic sauce
- 1 tablespoon sesame oil infused with garlic
- 1 tablespoon ginger, fresh, grated
- 1 tablespoon garlic, minced
- 1 red onion, cut into quarters and separated by petals
- 2 cups bell peppers, red, green, yellow
- 1 can whole water chestnuts, cut in half

- ½ pound fresh mushrooms halved
- 32 oz. boneless tuna, chunks or steaks
- 1 Splenda packet
- 2 zucchini, sliced
- 1 inch thick, keep skins on

Directions

1. Layer the tuna and the vegetable pieces evenly onto 8 skewers.
2. Combine the spices and the oil and chili sauce, add the Splenda
3. Quickly blend, either in a blender or by Quickly whipping.
4. Brush onto the kabob pieces, make sure every piece is coated
5. Grill 4 minutes on each side, check to ensure the tuna is cooked to taste.
6. Serving size is two skewers.
7. Mix the marinade ingredients and store in a covered container in the fridge. Place all the vegetables in one container in the fridge.
8. Place the tuna in a separate zip-lock bag.

Nutritional Value:

Calories: 467,

Total Fat: 18g,

Protein: 56g,

Total Carbs: 21g,

Dietary Fiber: 3.5g,

Sugar: 6g,

Sodium: 433mg

Chicken Relleno Casserole

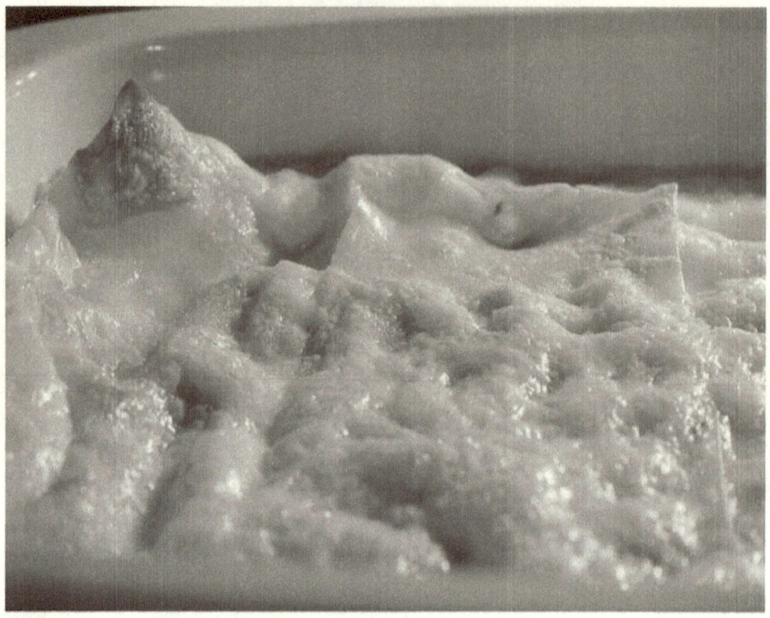

Prep time: 19 minutes

Cook time: 29 minutes

Number of Servings: 4

Ingredients

- 6 Tortilla Factory low-carb whole wheat tortillas, torn into small pieces
- 1 ½ cups hand-shredded cheese, Mexican
- 1 beaten egg
- 1 cup milk
- 2 cups cooked chicken, shredded
- 1 can Ro-tel
- ½ cup salsa verde

Directions

1. Grease an 8 x 8 glass baking dish

2. Heat oven to 375 degrees

3. Combine everything, but reserve ½ cup of the cheese

4. Bake it for 29 minutes

5. Take it out of the oven and add ½ cup cheese

6. Broil for about 2 minutes to melt the cheese

7. Let the casserole cool. Slice into 6 pieces and place in freezer containers, (1 cup with a lid) Freeze. Microwave for 2 minutes to serve. Top with sour cream, if desired.

Nutritional Value:

Calories: 265,

Total Fat: 16g,

Protein: 20g,

Total Carbs: 18g,

Dietary Fiber: 10g,

Sugar: 0g,

Sodium: 708mg

Steak Salad with Asian Spice

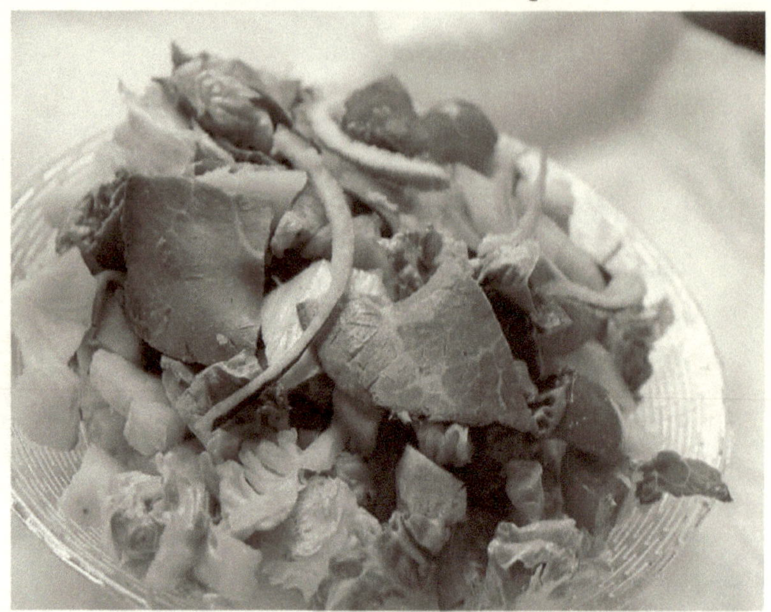

Prep time: 4 minutes

Cook time: 4 minutes

Number of Servings: 2

Ingredients

- 2 tablespoon sriracha sauce
- 1 tablespoon garlic, minced
- 1 tablespoon ginger, fresh, grated
- 1 bell pepper, yellow, cut into thin strips
- 1 bell pepper, red, cut into thin strips
- 1 tablespoon sesame oil, garlic
- 1 Splenda packet
- ½ tablespoon curry powder
- ½ tablespoon rice wine vinegar

- 8 oz. of beef sirloin, cut into strips
- 2 cups baby spinach, stemmed
- ½ head butter lettuce, torn or chopped into bite-sized pieces

Directions

1. Place the garlic, sriracha sauce, 1 tablespoon sesame oil, rice wine vinegar, and Splenda into a bowl and combine well.
2. Pour half of this mix into a zip-lock bag. Add the steak to marinade while you are preparing the salad.
3. Assemble the brightly colored salad by layering in two bowls.
4. Place the baby spinach into the bottom of the bowl. Place the butter lettuce next.
5. Mix the two peppers and place on top.
6. Remove the steak from the marinade and discard the liquid and bag.
7. Heat the sesame oil and quickly stir fry the steak until desired doneness, it should take about 3 minutes.
8. Place the steak on top of the salad.
9. Drizzle with the remaining dressing (another half of marinade mix).
10. Sprinkle sriracha sauce across the salad.
11. Combine the salad ingredients and place in a zip-lock bag in the fridge. Mix the marinade and halve into 2 zip-lock bags. Place the sriracha sauce into a small sealed container. Slice the steak and freeze in a zip-lock bag with the marinade. To prepare, mix the ingredients like the initial directions. Stir fry the marinated beef for 4 minutes to take into consideration the beef is frozen.

Nutritional Value:

Calories: 350,

Total Fat: 23g,

Protein: 28g,

Total Carbs: 7g,

Dietary Fiber: 3.5,

Sugar: 0,

Sodium: 267mg

Chicken Chow Mein Stir Fry

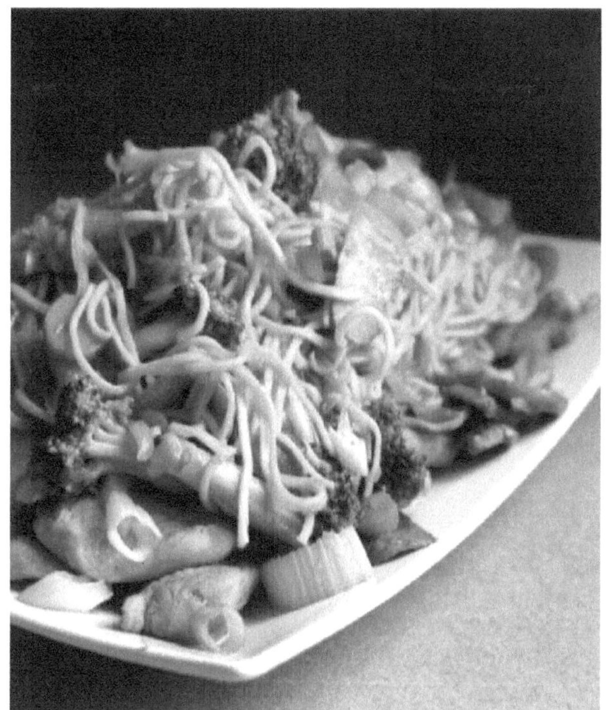

Prep time: 9 minutes

Cook time: 14 minutes

Number of Servings: 4

Ingredients

- 1/2 cup sliced onion
- 2 tablespoon Oil, sesame garlic flavored
- 4 cups shredded Bok-Choy
- 1 cup Sugar Snap Peas
- 1 cup fresh bean sprouts
- 3 stalks Celery, chopped
- 1 1/2 tablespoon minced Garlic

- 1 packet Splenda
- 1 cup Broth, chicken
- 2 tablespoon Soy Sauce
- 1 tablespoon ginger, freshly minced
- 1 tablespoon cornstarch
- 4 boneless Chicken Breasts, cooked/sliced thinly

Directions

1. Place the bok-choy, peas, celery in a skillet with 1 T garlic oil.
2. Stir fry until bok-choy is softened to liking.
3. Add remaining ingredients except for the cornstarch.
4. If too thin, stir cornstarch into ½ cup cold water when smooth pour into skillet.
5. Bring cornstarch and chow mein to a one-minute boil. Turn off the heat source.
6. Stir sauce then wait for 4 minutes to serve, after the chow mein has thickened.
7. Freeze in covered containers. Heat for 2 minutes in the microwave before serving.

Nutritional Value:

Calories: 368,

Total Fat: 18g,

Protein: 42g,

Total Carbs: 12g,

Dietary Fiber: 16g,

Sugar: 6g,

Sodium: 746mg

Salmon with Bok-Choy

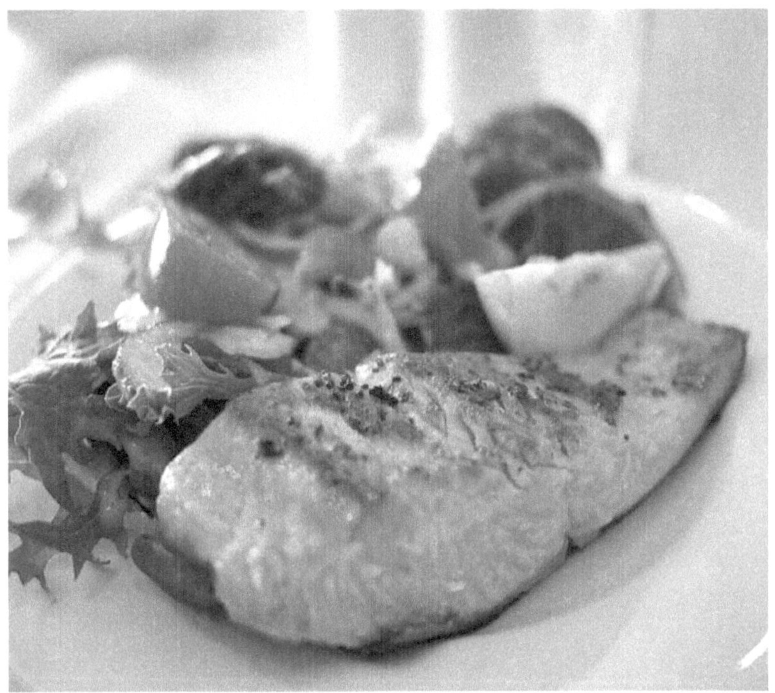

Prep time: 9 minutes

Cook time: 9 minutes

Number of Servings: 4

Ingredients

- 1 cup red peppers, roasted, drained
- 2 cups chopped bok-choy
- 1 tablespoon salted butter
- 5 oz. salmon steak
- 1 lemon, sliced very thinly
- 1/8 tablespoon black pepper
- 1 tablespoon olive oil

- 2 tablespoon sriracha sauce

Directions

1. Place oil in a skillet
2. Place all but 4 slices of lemon in the skillet.
3. Sprinkle the bok choy with the black pepper.
4. Stir fry the bok-choy with the lemons.
5. Remove and place on four plates.
6. Place the butter in the skillet and stir fry the salmon, turning once.
7. Place the salmon on the bed of bok-choy.
8. Divide the red peppers and encircle the salmon.
9. Place a slice of lemon atop the salmon.
10. Drizzle with sriracha sauce.
11. Freeze the cooked salmon in individual zip-lock bags. Place the bok-choy, with the remaining ingredients into one-cup containers. Microwave the salmon for one minute and the frozen bok choy for two. Assemble to serve.

Nutritional Value:

Calories: 410,

Total Fat: 30g,

Protein: 30g,

Total Carbs: 7g,

Dietary Fiber: 2g,

Sugar: 0g,

Sodium: 200mg

Soups & Stews

Cream Zucchini Soup

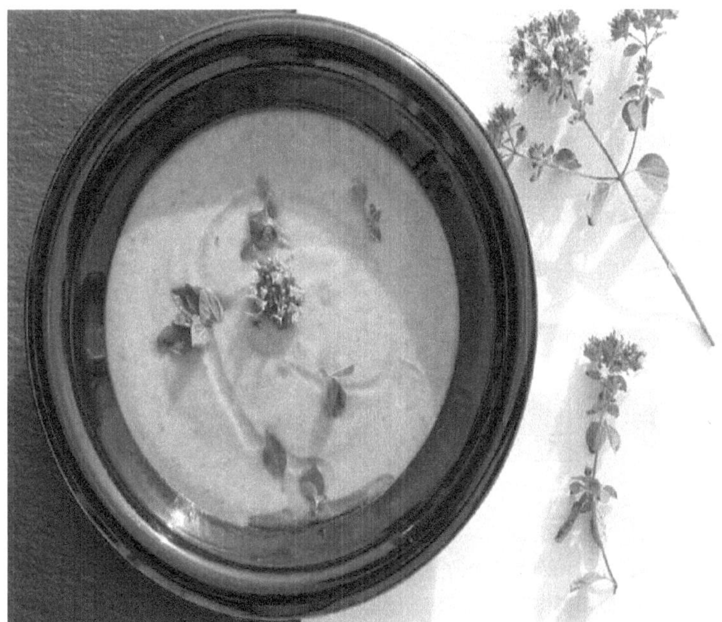

Prep Time: 8-10 min.

Cooking Time: 8 min.

Number of Servings: 4

Ingredients:

- 2 cups vegetable stock
- 2 garlic cloves, crushed
- 1 tablespoon butter
- 4 (preferably medium size) zucchinis, peeled and chopped
- 1 small onion, chopped
- 2 cups heavy cream
- 1/2 teaspoon dried oregano, (finely ground)
- 1/2 teaspoon black pepper, (finely ground)
- 1 teaspoon dried parsley, (finely ground)
- 1 teaspoon of sea salt

- Lemon juice (optional)

Directions:

1. Arrange Instant Pot over a dry platform in your kitchen. Open its top lid and switch it on.
2. Find and press "SAUTE" cooking function; add the butter in it and allow it to melt.
3. In the pot, add the onions, zucchini, garlic; cook (while stirring) until turns translucent and softened for around 2-3 minutes.
4. Add the vegetable broth and sprinkle with salt, oregano, pepper, and parsley; gently stir to mix well.
5. Close the lid to create a locked chamber; make sure that safety valve is in locking position.
6. Find and press "MANUAL" cooking function; timer to 5 minutes with default "HIGH" pressure mode.
7. Allow the pressure to build to cook the ingredients.
8. After cooking time is over press "CANCEL" setting. Find and press "QPR" cooking function. This setting is for quick release of inside pressure.
9. Slowly open the lid, take out the cooked recipe in serving plates or serving bowls, and enjoy the keto recipe. Top with some lemon juice.

Nutritional Values (Per Serving):

Calories - 264

Fat – 26g

Saturated Fat – 7g

Trans Fat – 0g

Carbohydrates – 11g

Fiber – 3g

Sodium – 564mg

Protein – 4g

Coconut Chicken Soup

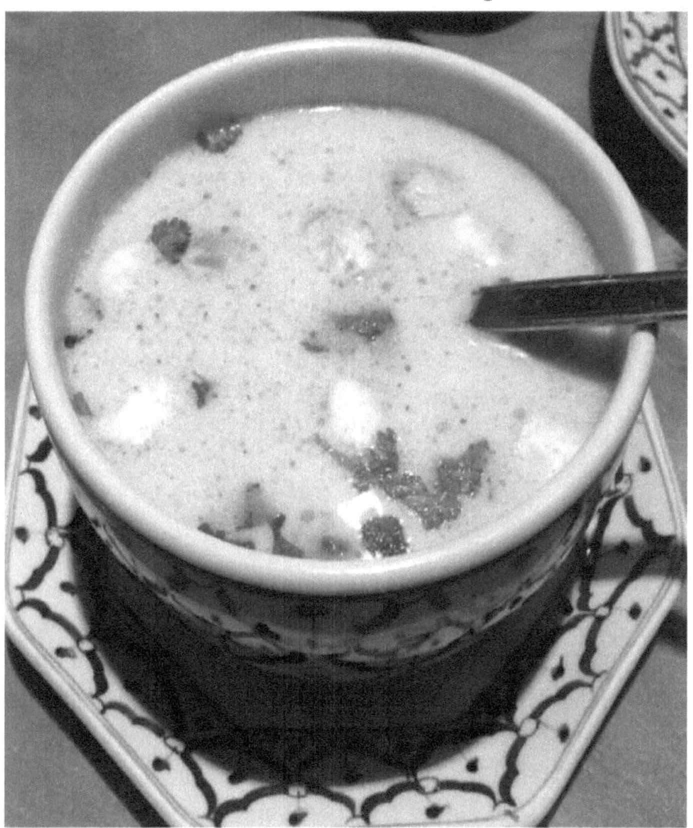

Prep Time: 8-10 min.

Cooking Time: 18 min.

Number of Servings: 4

Ingredients:

- 4 cloves of garlic, minced
- 1 pound chicken breasts, skin-on
- 4 cups of water
- 2 tablespoons olive oil
- 1 onion, diced
- 1 cup of coconut milk
- (finely ground) black pepper and salt as per taste preference

- 2 tablespoons sesame oil

Directions:

1. Arrange Instant Pot over a dry platform in your kitchen. Open its top lid and switch it on.
2. Find and press "SAUTE" cooking function; add the oil in it and allow it to heat.
3. In the pot, add the onions, garlic; cook (while stirring) until turns translucent and softened for around 1-2 minutes.
4. Stir in the chicken breasts; stir, and cook for 2 more minutes.
5. Pour in water and coconut milk — season to taste.
6. Close the lid to create a locked chamber; make sure that safety valve is in locking position.
7. Find and press "MANUAL" cooking function; timer to 15 minutes with default "HIGH" pressure mode.
8. Allow the pressure to build to cook the ingredients.
9. After cooking time is over press "CANCEL" setting. Find and press "NPR" cooking function. This setting is for the natural release of inside pressure and it takes around 10 minutes to slowly release pressure.
10. Slowly open the lid, Drizzle with sesame oil on top.
11. Take out the cooked recipe in serving plates or serving bowls and enjoy the keto recipe.

Nutritional Values (Per Serving):

Calories - 328

Fat – 31g

Saturated Fat – 6g

Trans Fat – 0g

Carbohydrates – 6g

Fiber – 4g

Sodium – 76mg

Protein – 21g

Chicken Bacon Soup

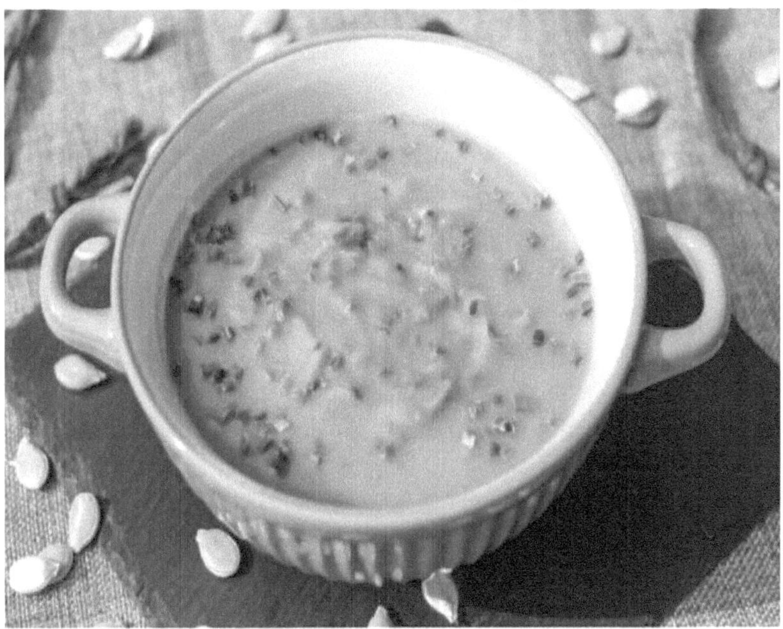

Prep Time: 8-10 min.

Cooking Time: 40 min.

Number of Servings: 4

Ingredients:

- 6 boneless, skinless chicken thighs, make cubes
- ½ cup chopped celery
- 4 minced garlic cloves
- 6-ounce mushrooms, sliced
- ½ cup chopped onion
- 8-ounce softened cream cheese
- ¼ cup softened butter
- 1 teaspoon dried thyme
- Salt and (finely ground) black pepper, as per taste preference
- 2 cups chopped spinach
- 8 ounces cooked bacon slices, chopped
- 3 cups (preferably homemade) chicken broth

- 1 cup heavy cream

Directions:

1. Arrange Instant Pot over a dry platform in your kitchen. Open its top lid and switch it on.
2. Add the ingredients except for the cream, spinach, and bacon; gently stir to mix well.
3. Close the lid to create a locked chamber; make sure that safety valve is in locking position.
4. Find and press "SOUP" cooking function; timer to 30 minutes with default "HIGH" pressure mode.
5. Allow the pressure to build to cook the ingredients.
6. After cooking time is over press "CANCEL" setting. Find and press "NPR" cooking function. This setting is for the natural release of inside pressure and it takes around 10 minutes to slowly release pressure.
7. Slowly open the lid, stir in cream and spinach.
8. Take out the cooked recipe in serving plates or serving bowls and enjoy the keto recipe. Top with the bacon.

Nutritional Values (Per Serving):

Calories - 456

Fat – 38g

Saturated Fat – 13g

Trans Fat – 0g

Carbohydrates – 7g

Fiber – 1g

Sodium – 742mg

Protein – 23g

Cream Pepper Stew

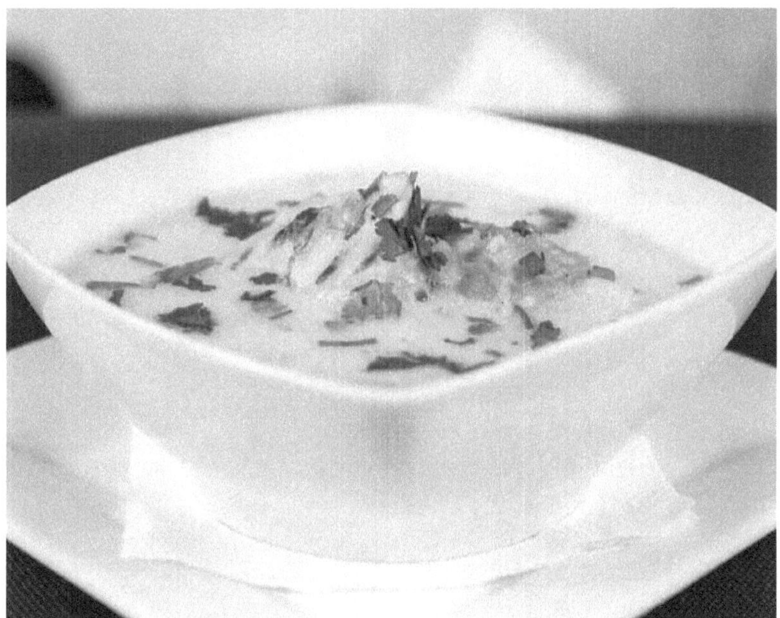

Prep Time: 8-10 min.

Cooking Time: 10 min.

Number of Servings: 4

Ingredients:

- 1 (preferably medium size) celery stalk, chopped
- 1 (preferably medium size) yellow bell pepper, chopped
- 1 (preferably medium size) green bell pepper, chopped
- 2 large red bell peppers, chopped
- 1 small red onion, chopped
- 2 tablespoons butter
- 1/2 cup cream cheese, full-fat
- 1/4 teaspoon dried thyme, (finely ground)
- 1/2 teaspoon black pepper, (finely ground)
- 1 teaspoon dried parsley, (finely ground)
- 1 teaspoon salt
- 2 cups vegetable stock

- 1 cup heavy cream

Directions:

1. Arrange Instant Pot over a dry platform in your kitchen. Open its top lid and switch it on.
2. Find and press "SAUTE" cooking function; add the butter in it and allow it to heat.
3. In the pot, add the onions, bell pepper, and celery; cook (while stirring) until turns translucent and softened for around 3-4 minutes.
4. Pour in the vegetable stock and heavy cream — season with salt, pepper, parsley, and thyme.
5. Close the lid to create a locked chamber; make sure that safety valve is in locking position.
6. Find and press "MANUAL" cooking function; timer to 6 minutes with default "HIGH" pressure mode.
7. Allow the pressure to build to cook the ingredients.
8. After cooking time is over press "CANCEL" setting. Find and press "QPR" cooking function. This setting is for quick release of inside pressure.
9. Slowly open the lid, mix in the cream; take out the cooked recipe in serving plates or serving bowls, and enjoy the keto recipe.

Nutritional Values (Per Serving):

Calories - 286

Fat – 27g

Saturated Fat – 6g

Trans Fat – 0g

Carbohydrates – 9g

Fiber – 3g

Sodium – 523mg

Protein – 5g

Ham Asparagus Soup

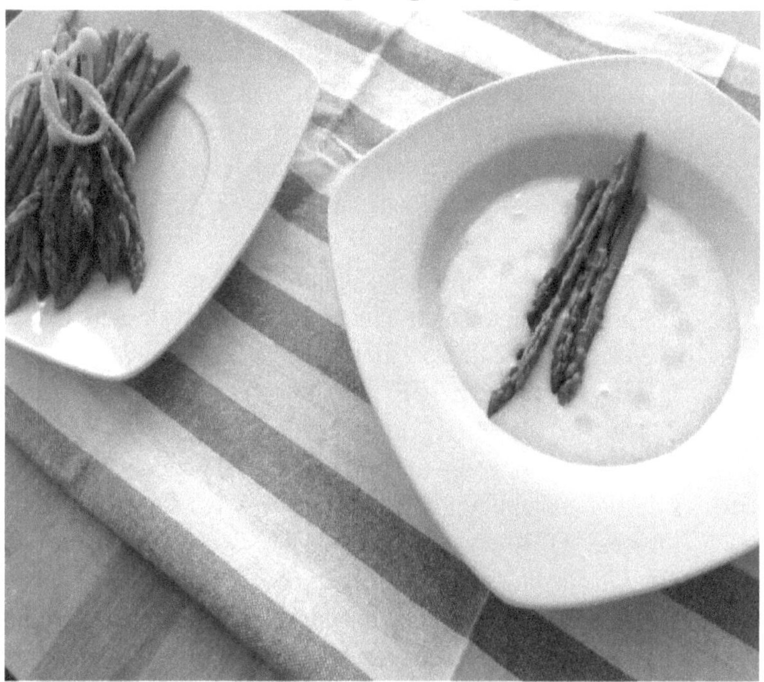

Prep Time: 8-10 min.

Cooking Time: 55 min.

Number of Servings: 3-4

Ingredients:

- 5 crushed garlic cloves
- 1 cup chopped ham
- 4 cups (preferably homemade) chicken broth
- 2 pounds trimmed and halved asparagus spears
- 2 tablespoons butter
- 1 chopped yellow onion
- ½ teaspoon dried thyme
- Salt and freshly (finely ground) black pepper, as per taste preference

Directions:

1. Arrange Instant Pot over a dry platform in your kitchen. Open its top lid and switch it on.
2. Find and press "SAUTE" cooking function; add the butter in it and allow it to heat.
3. In the pot, add the onions; cook (while stirring) until turns translucent and softened for around 4-5 minutes.
4. Add the garlic, ham bone and broth; stir, and cook for about 2-3 minutes.
5. Add the other ingredients; gently stir to mix well.
6. Close the lid to create a locked chamber; make sure that safety valve is in locking position.
7. Find and press "SOUP" cooking function; timer to 45 minutes with default "HIGH" pressure mode.
8. Allow the pressure to build to cook the ingredients.
9. After cooking time is over press "CANCEL" setting. Find and press "QPR" cooking function. This setting is for quick release of inside pressure.
10. Slowly open the lid, add the prepared recipe mix in a blender or processor.
11. Blend or process to make a smooth mix. Place the mix in serving bowls and enjoy the keto recipe.

Nutritional Values (Per Serving):

Calories - 146

Fat – 7g

Saturated Fat – 3g

Trans Fat – 0g

Carbohydrates – 5g

Fiber – 4g

Sodium – 262mg

Protein – 10g

Delicious Desserts

Almond Mug Cake

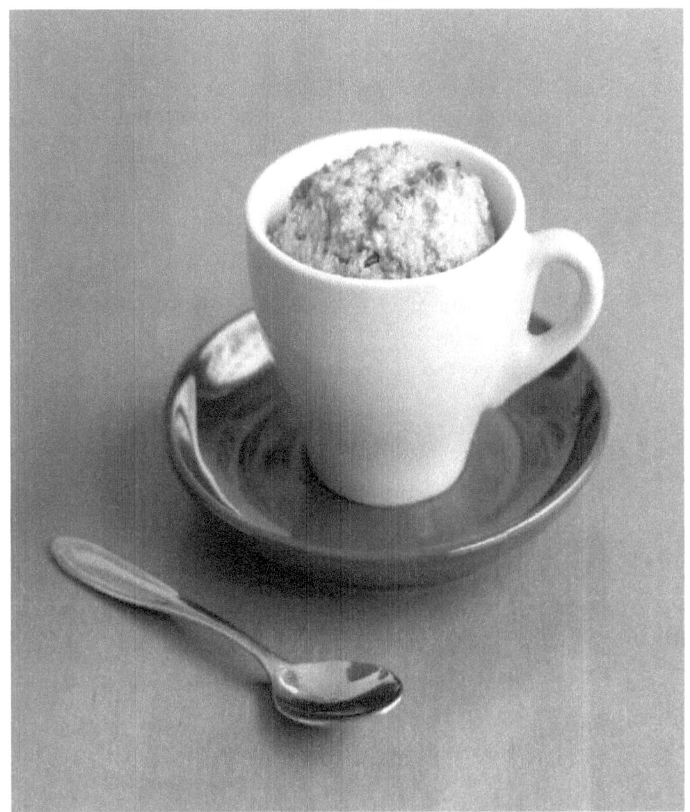

Prep Time: 8-10 min.

Cooking Time: 10 min.

Number of Servings: 1

Ingredients:

- 1/4 teaspoon baking powder
- 1/4 teaspoon vanilla extract
- 1 1/2 tablespoons cacao powder
- 1 egg, beaten
- 1/4 cup almond flour

- 1 teaspoon cinnamon powder
- 2 tablespoons stevia powder
- A pinch of salt

Directions:

1. Combine all ingredients in the bowl until well-combined. Add the mix in a heat-proof mug; cover with a foil.
2. Arrange Instant Pot over a dry platform in your kitchen. Open its top lid and switch it on.
3. In the pot, pour water. Arrange a trivet or steamer basket inside that came with Instant Pot. Now place/arrange the mug over the trivet/basket.
4. Close the lid to create a locked chamber; make sure that safety valve is in locking position.
5. Find and press "MANUAL" cooking function; timer to 10 minutes with default "HIGH" pressure mode.
6. Allow the pressure to build to cook the ingredients.
7. After cooking time is over press "CANCEL" setting. Find and press "QPR" cooking function. This setting is for quick release of inside pressure.
8. Slowly open the lid, cool down the mug, and serve warm.

Nutritional Values (Per Serving):

Calories - 138

Fat – 13g

Saturated Fat – 6g

Trans Fat – 0g

Carbohydrates – 7g

Fiber – 3g

Sodium – 73mg

Protein – 9g

Tapioca Keto Pudding

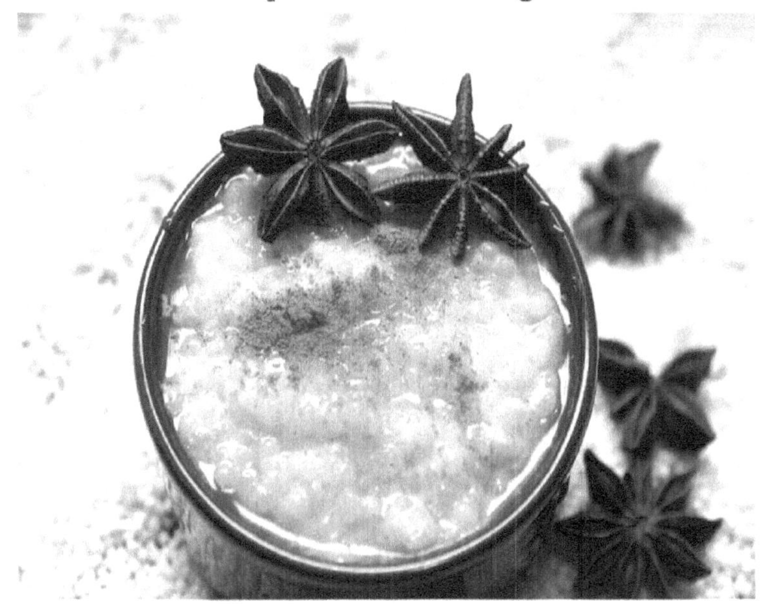

Prep Time: 8-10 min.

Cooking Time: 20 min.

Number of Servings: 4

Ingredients:

- 1 tablespoon Erythritol
- 1 teaspoon chia seeds
- 1 tablespoon tapioca
- 1 tablespoon butter
- 2 cup heavy cream
- 1/4 cup raspberries or strawberries, mashed

Directions:

1. Arrange Instant Pot over a dry platform in your kitchen. Open its top lid and switch it on.
2. Find and press "SAUTE" cooking function.
3. In the pot, add the cream; cook (while stirring) for 4-5

minutes.

4. Add the tapioca and stir it well. Add the Erythritol and butter.
5. In a bowl, mix the chia seeds and berries.
6. Add the berry mix in the pot and stir well.
7. Close the lid to create a locked chamber; make sure that safety valve is in locking position.
8. Find and press "MANUAL" cooking function; timer to 15 minutes with default "HIGH" pressure mode.
9. Allow the pressure to build to cook the ingredients.
10. After cooking time is over press "CANCEL" setting. Find and press "QPR" cooking function. This setting is for quick release of inside pressure.
11. Add in serving bowls, cool down and place in the fridge for 2 hours.
12. Serve chilled.

Nutritional Values (Per Serving):

Calories - 246

Fat – 24g

Saturated Fat – 9g

Trans Fat – 0g

Carbohydrates – 10g

Fiber – 2g

Sodium – 183mg

Protein – 3g

Cream Chocolate Delight

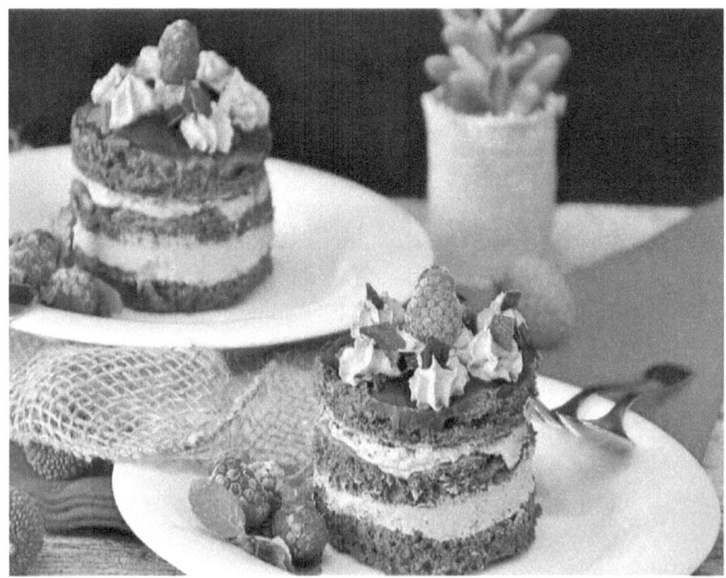

Prep Time: 8-10 min.

Cooking Time: 15 min.

Number of Servings: 4

Ingredients:

- 1 teaspoon orange zest
- 1 teaspoon stevia powder
- 2 heavy cream
- ¼ cup unsweetened dark chocolate, chopped
- 3 eggs
- 1 teaspoon vanilla extract
- ½ teaspoon salt

Directions:

1. Arrange Instant Pot over a dry platform in your kitchen. Open its top lid and switch it on.
2. Find and press "SAUTE" cooking function.
3. In the pot, add the heavy cream, chopped chocolate, stevia

powder, vanilla extract, orange zest, and salt; cook (while stirring) until the chocolate is melted.

4. Crack eggs in the pot; stirring constantly. Remove from the instant pot. Add the mixture to 4 mason jars with loose lids.
5. In the pot, pour water. Arrange a trivet or steamer basket inside that came with Instant Pot. Now place/arrange the jars over the trivet/basket.
6. Close the lid to create a locked chamber; make sure that safety valve is in locking position.
7. Find and press "MANUAL" cooking function; timer to 10 minutes with default "HIGH" pressure mode.
8. Allow the pressure to build to cook the ingredients.
9. After cooking time is over press "CANCEL" setting. Find and press "QPR" cooking function. This setting is for quick release of inside pressure.
10. Slowly open the lid, cool down the jars, and chill in the fridge. Serve chilled.

Nutritional Values (Per Serving):

Calories - 254

Fat – 26g

Saturated Fat – 12g

Trans Fat – 0g

Carbohydrates – 5g

Fiber – 1g

Sodium – 168mg

Protein – 8g

Coconut Keto Pudding

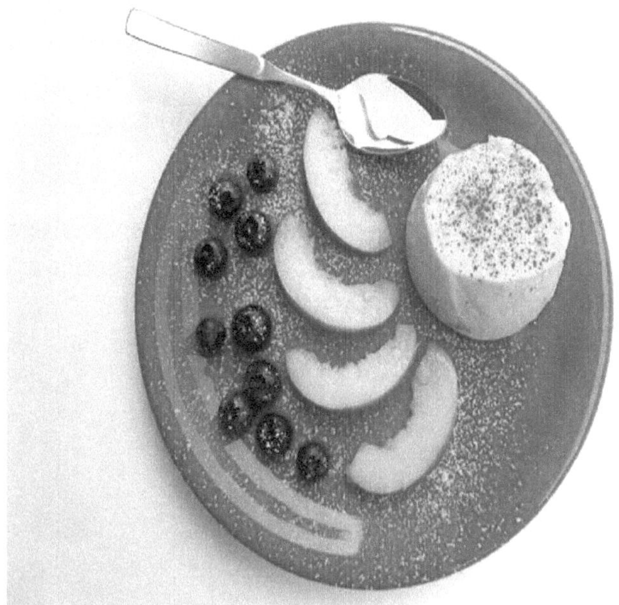

Prep Time: 8-10 min.

Cooking Time: 5 min.

Number of Servings: 4

Ingredients:

- 3 tablespoons Stevia granular
- 1/2 teaspoon vanilla extract
- 1 2/3 cup coconut milk
- 3 egg yolks
- 1 tablespoon gelatin

Directions:

1. Arrange Instant Pot over a dry platform in your kitchen. Open its top lid and switch it on.
2. Add the coconut milk.
3. Close the lid to create a locked chamber; make sure that safety

valve is in locking position.

4. Find and press "MANUAL" cooking function; timer to 5 minutes with default "HIGH" pressure mode.
5. Allow the pressure to build to cook the ingredients.
6. After cooking time is over press "CANCEL" setting. Find and press "QPR" cooking function. This setting is for quick release of inside pressure.
7. Place the coconut milk in the Instant Pot. Close the lid and make sure that the steam release valve is set to "Sealing."
8. Whisk in egg yolks and the rest of the ingredients.
9. Find and press "SAUTE" cooking function. Cook until boiling the mix.
10.   Add in serving bowls, cool down and place in the fridge for 2 hours.
11.   Serve chilled.

Nutritional Values (Per Serving):

Calories - 246

Fat – 27g

Saturated Fat – 8g

Trans Fat – 0g

Carbohydrates – 7g

Fiber – 4g

Sodium – 89mg

Protein – 4g

Vanilla Cream Delight

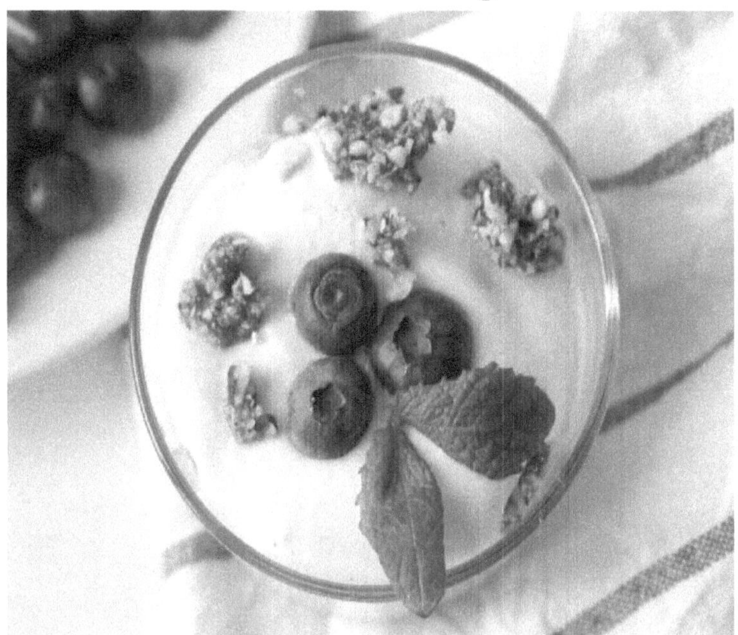

Prep Time: 8-10 min.

Cooking Time: 15 min.

Number of Servings: 4

Ingredients:

- 1 ½ cup heavy cream
- 1 teaspoon vanilla extract
- 8 large eggs
- ¾ cup unsweetened almond milk
- 1 vanilla bean
- 4 tablespoons stevia granular

Directions:

1. Cut the vanilla bean lengthwise using a knife and take out the seeds. Add in a mixing bowl.
2. Mix in the remaining ingredients. Whisk the mix thoroughly

and add into four ramekins.

3. Arrange Instant Pot over a dry platform in your kitchen. Open its top lid and switch it on.
4. In the pot, pour 2 cups water. Arrange a trivet or steamer basket inside that came with Instant Pot. Now place/arrange the ramekins over the trivet/basket.
5. Close the lid to create a locked chamber; make sure that safety valve is in locking position.
6. Find and press "MANUAL" cooking function; timer to 15 minutes with default "HIGH" pressure mode.
7. Allow the pressure to build to cook the ingredients.
8. After cooking time is over press "CANCEL" setting. Find and press "QPR" cooking function. This setting is for quick release of inside pressure.
9. Slowly open the lid, cool down the ramekins.
10. Chill in fridge and serve.

Nutritional Values (Per Serving):

Calories - 318

Fat – 26g

Saturated Fat – 7g

Trans Fat – 0g

Carbohydrates – 3g

Fiber – 0g

Sodium – 106mg

Protein – 13g

Conclusion

That is pretty much it. With this knowledge, you should be able to jump on the keto diet wagon without worry. As with anything else in the health and lifestyle field, make sure to consult your doctor or dietitian first before you try out any new diet. That applies to the keto diet as well. While other people may be successful with their weight-loss endeavor with this diet, you may fail simply because your body reacts differently.

Remember that consistency is key. A keto diet can be difficult for some people, but keep at it long enough and you will come to enjoy it. You will lose weight, become fit and the envy of your fellow friends.

With all of that said and done, I wish you the very best in your health and lifestyle endeavor.